Pediatric Orthopedics for Primary Care Physicians

This revised and extended new edition retains the features that made the first edition such a popular text for pediatricians and primary care physicians: orthopedic disorders are arranged according to age of onset and also according to their frequency of occurrence, and this is supplemented with helpful guidelines for orthopedic referral. Distilling a vast wealth of the author's experience in this area, the book provides a user-friendly, concise, and readable account of all the main pediatric orthopedic complications, with the addition in this new edition of helpful "pearl" boxes to highlight salient features of the given disorder. A new chapter on the genetics of these disorders provides additional useful background. The new edition is also richly illustrated throughout with many new radiographs and line drawings to supplement the text.

Written specifically for residents and attending physicians in pediatrics and family practice, this volume will help doctors provide the optimal care for these patients.

DENNIS S. WEINER, M.D. is Chairman of Pediatric Orthopaedic Surgery at the Children's Hospital Medical Center of Akron, Ohio, where he is also Director of Orthopaedic Research. He is also Professor of Orthopaedics at the Northeastern Ohio Universities College of Medicine.

PEDIATRIC ORTHOPEDICS

for Primary Care Physicians

Second Edition

Dennis S. Weiner, M.D.

Children's Hospital Medical Center of Akron
AK, Ohio, USA

Northeastern Ohio Universities College of
Medicine – Rootstown, Ohio, USA

Assistant Editor

Kerwyn Jones, M.D.

Children's Hospital Medical Center of Akron
AK, Ohio, USA

Northeastern Ohio Universities College of
Medicine – Rootstown, Ohio, USA

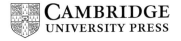

PUBLISHED BY THE PRESS SYNDICATE OF THE UNIVERSITY OF CAMBRIDGE
The Pitt Building, Trumpington Street, Cambridge, United Kingdom

CAMBRIDGE UNIVERSITY PRESS
The Edinburgh Building, Cambridge CB2 2RU, UK
40 West 20th Street, New York, NY 10011–4211, USA
477 Williamstown Road, Port Melbourne, VIC 3207, Australia
Ruiz de Alarcón 13, 28014 Madrid, Spain
Dock House, The Waterfront, Cape Town 8001, South Africa

http://www.cambridge.org

First edition © Churchill Livingstone 1993
Second edition © Cambridge University Press 2004

First published by Churchill Livingstone, 1993
Second edition 2004

Printed in the United Kingdom at the University Press, Cambridge

Typefaces Utopia 9/13 pt. and Formata   *System* $\mathrm{\LaTeX\,2_\varepsilon}$ [TB]

A catalog record for this book is available from the British Library

ISBN 0 521 82564 4 hardback

To my wife, Phyllis Ann Weiner, whose unfailing patience, understanding, support, and sacrifice has fostered its genesis, and to our children, Scott, Tracy, Brad, Kristin, Timothy, Sherri and Romy.

To Dr. Ian Macnab, my revered mentor, the catalyst and stimulant of this effort, for the years of his scholarly advice and the brilliance of his teaching.

To Dr. Harry W. Odell, my esteemed training chief; and to my parents, Milt and Adeline, for the nurturing that allowed this to take form and shape, and especially my mother Adeline, the most loving and lovable person I have ever known.

Contents

6   Miscellaneous disorders   115

Contributors

Scott D. Weiner, M.D.
Director of Resident Education and Assistant
Chairman of Orthopaedics, Division Chief of
Oncology, Summa Health Systems-Akron, Ohio, USA
Consultant Pediatric Orthopaedics Oncology,
Children's Hospital Medical Center of Akron-Akron,
Ohio, USA
Associate Professor of Orthopaedic Surgery,
Northeastern Ohio Universities College of
Medicine – Rootstown, Ohio, USA

Bradley K. Weiner, M.D.
Associate Professor and Director of the Spine Unit,
Pennsylvania State University – Hershey,
Pennsylvania, USA
Adult Spine Consultant, Regional Skeletal Dysplasia
Center, Children's Hospital Medical Center of
Akron – Akron, Ohio, USA
Staff Orthopaedic Surgeon, Children's Hospital
Medical Center of Akron – Akron, Ohio, USA
Assistant Professor of Orthopaedic Surgery,
Northeastern Ohio, USA Universities College of
Medicine – Rootstown, Ohio, USA

Foreword

The style of this book is unique in the medical literature. It reads like a novel, yet teaches forcibly. It is a pleasure to be able to learn while sitting comfortably in an armchair. It discusses patients – not diseases. It describes the child who limps into the office, and answers the question, "What is the cause of this limp, and how should I treat it?" Of equal importance, it describes the cases that are normal variants, for which treatment is not necessary. These sections are crucial because they point out the difference between adult orthopedics and pediatric orthopedics. In adult orthopedics, the patient needs a detailed explanation, a clear description of the treatment considered necessary and the results that can be reasonably anticipated. In pediatric orthopedics, the same detailed explanation should and *must* be given to the parents.

Certain children should be sent for a second opinion and, if necessary, for treatment by the surgeon whose opinion has been sought. The text clearly indicates the reasons for this approach.

Dennis Weiner is well known for his detailed knowledge of orthopedic pathology and his special skills in carrying out surgical corrections when necessary. This book is not cluttered, however, with a description of surgical minutiae.

This is a book that was waiting to be written, a fact that is amply demonstrated by both the text and the diagrams.

I would like to commend this book and to congratulate Dennis Weiner for carrying out the responsibility in a magnificent manner. This book will be a classic in its own time.

Ian Macnab

M.B., Ch.B., F.R.C.S. (England), F.R.C.S.

Professor Emeritus, Department of Orthopaedic
   Surgery,

University of Toronto Faculty of Medicine, Toronto,
   Ontario, Canada

Preface to first edition

This book is in large part dedicated to the many pediatric, family practice and orthopedic residents who have enriched my personal education as they have moved through their pediatric orthopedic rotations, during which I served as their mentor. It is also, clearly, the culmination of their individual inquisitiveness and their perspicacity in continually challenging our traditional views of the treatment for common orthopedic problems. Many of these conditions have now been discovered to have rather innocuous natural evolutions if left totally unattended. It is, in fact, a sorry commentary to relate that many patients would have been far better off to have "rubbed a potato" on their head three times a day rather than having ever seen a medical practitioner for their complaints. These residents' questions have provided the stimulus for this author to consolidate the available knowledge into a simplified, concise, and meaningful approach to the various conditions. Sorrowfully, the scope of our current knowledge of the natural history of many of these pediatric orthopedic disorders is still rather miniscule. It is, however, hoped that the material within aptly reflects our current level of understanding.

Ultimately, the ideal is that this book will inhabit a small space in the office and home libraries of all physicians caring for children and adolescents with bone and joint disorders. It is not intended as an encyclopedic compendium of differential diagnoses, but rather as a useful handbook that attempts to crystallize in concise form the characterization of a given condition.

The presentation of the material is being offered in a somewhat untraditional fashion; namely, in order of the frequency or rarity by which these conditions will likely be encountered in a practice situation, and more importantly, by the age at which the conditions would most commonly present for medical attention.

Preface to second edition

The reader of this second edition of "Pediatric Orthopedics for Primary Care Physicians" will hopefully be favorably impressed by the addition of a current update to all chapters in the book and particularly the addition of "pearl" boxes highlighting the salient features of the given disorders. Additionally a chapter on genetics in orthopedic conditions has been added. The entire content of the book has been reviewed and updated to the date of publication. It is hoped by the author that this current edition will provide a useful resource for all primary care physicians seeing children with orthopedic problems.

Acknowledgments

I wish to express my sincerest gratitude to Mr. Tom Campbell for a yeoman effort in medical illustration and visual reproduction, and the entire Audio-Visual Department at Children's Hospital Medical Center of Akron; Mrs. Allison Allen for clerical and typographical assistance of a monumental nature; Mrs. Bonnie Leighley for project coordination; Dr. Kerwyn Jones for critical review and updating of the text; Dr. Scott Weiner for his contribution in Chapter 6 on malignant soft tissue and bone lesions; Dr. Brad Weiner for his contribution in Chapter 5 on backache and disc disease; and to the many primary care physicians who helped catalyze this effort.

Chapter 1

Basic considerations in growing bones and joints

A mind that can comprehend the principles, will devise its own methods.

N. Andry, *Orthopaedia*, 1783.

The growth plate

Although there are clear and distinct structural differences between very young and mature bones, the structure that most clearly separates them is the physis or growth plate. Anatomically situated beneath the epiphysis and above the metaphysis and diaphysis, its role in our maturing process is a noble work of nature. Not only does it afford us eventual height and body mass, it contributes to our necessary resiliency and elasticity when we are mentally too young to avoid "leaping off high structures," "somersaulting," "performing backflips," and other such attempts to convert ourselves into unguarded flying missiles.

The upper cellular layer(s) of the growth plate are in a resting (germinal) stage, waiting to be converted into actively reproducing cells (chondrocytes) that will add to our eventual height by replicating in a longitudinal fashion (Figure 1.1). These cells also are responsible for producing the matrix in which they are embedded, most particularly the collagen that binds to the protein polysaccharide produced by these cells. This *zone of proliferation* is best conceived as an anabolic zone, where positive events are happening, both to elongate our bones and to build strength for the growth plate apparatus. Its tightly bound cells and matrix allow for considerable resistance to stress. The

Figure 1.1. The anatomic components of the physis (growth plate).

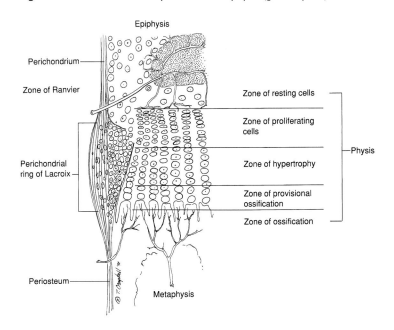

Epiphysis

Perichondrium

Zone of Ranvier

Zone of resting cells

Zone of proliferating cells

Physis

Zone of hypertrophy

Perichondrial ring of Lacroix

Zone of provisional ossification

Zone of ossification

Periosteum

Metaphysis

next zone closer to the metaphysis is the *zone of hypertrophy*. This zone is much more catabolic in nature, where preparations for the eventual conversion of growth plate cartilage into bone are occurring. The tightly packed linear oriented cells seen in the proliferative zone have now become swollen, and are surrounded by abundant matrix in which the collagen bundles are much more loosely and irregularly arranged. Catabolic enzyme activity predominates and the growth plate strength is weakest in this area. An intrinsic mechanism that has not been fully clarified, operates within the zone of hypertrophy that controls the programmed cellular "life to death" cycle of the chondroblast (apoptosis). Clinically this is the zone through which epiphyseal separations (fractures and slipped epiphyses) occur.

The lowest part of the zone of hypertrophy and the encroaching metaphyseal level is termed the *zone of provisional ossification*. The lower levels of the zone of hypertrophy are maturing and being converted into newly forming bone (osteoid). The most predominant anatomic structural difference in this region is the ingress of blood vessels carrying a high oxygen "front", which creates an environment in which cartilage cannot survive. By a process of cartilage removal and subsequent conversion into newly formed osteoid, the region begins to assume the characteristics seen in the upper layer of the metaphyseal region.

Two other commonly discussed structures have a profound bearing on growth plate integrity. The *zone of Ranvier* consists of cells lying laterally and circumferential around the upper zones of the physis whose responsibility it is to provide latitudinal growth of the physis and thereby provide for a wider bone at the level of the growth plate. The *perichondrial ring of Lacroix* is the continuation of the periosteum of the metaphysis as it reaches the growth plate to become the perichondrium of the epiphysis. This fibrocartilaginous osseous ring surrounds the growth plate, much like the

Birth

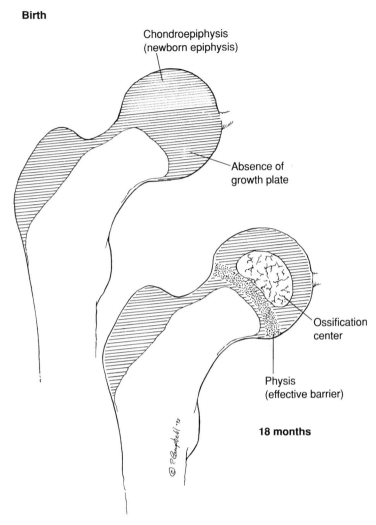

Chondroepiphysis
(newborn epiphysis)

Absence of
growth plate

Ossification
center

Physis
(effective barrier)

18 months

Figure 1.2. The configuration of the chondroepiphysis and its union with the greater trochanter in the neonate. This is contrasted with the presence of a secondary ossification center and an established growth plate as an effective barrier between the epiphysis and metaphysis, seen in the child between 12 and 24 months of age.

bark of a tree, and is believed to provide up to 50 percent of the resistance of the epiphysis to displacement.

The epiphysis, metaphysis, and diaphysis

The growth plate in newborns is not constituted as an effective structure between the metaphysis and the epiphysis, and this transformation generally does not occur until between 12 and 24 months of age (Figure 1.2).

Injury or disease affecting the metaphysis or epiphysis in the very young child (i.e. under one year of age) can often damage all elements of the growth plate apparatus spreading directly across from one zone to another. Once the growth plate is constituted, an effective barrier then develops between the epiphysis and metaphysis. The cartilage epiphysis prior to developing a primary center of ossification is termed a chondroepiphysis and is, as would be expected, less resistant to injury and disease. Its primary function is to evolve into an appropriate shape to provide a joint surface for motion and to be sturdy enough to absorb and transmit the loading stresses imposed on that joint. It also provides protection for the underlying growth plate.

The metaphysis is the most metabolically active area in growing bone, with the richest vascularity and the highest turnover of bone. The constant remodeling in this area allows for the internal reshaping of the bone in order to resist all manner of internal and external stresses. In a child, the large volume of cancellous bone compared with cortical bone in this region makes it obviously weaker than the cortical bone so prevalent in the diaphysis. For these accumulative reasons, bone pathology is most commonly reflected in the metaphysis (i.e., infection, tumors, and trauma).

The diaphysis is composed for the most part of cortical bone surrounding the medullary canal. Therefore, this region is much stronger, less elastic, and more protective in nature to provide resistance to the tremendous daily forces applied, and to keep us from "shattering." It must be remembered that the diaphysis also has a rich blood supply, and possesses periosteal and endosteal cells that can provide enormous amounts of new bone in times of stress (i.e., fracture).

Nutrition of bone

Bone possesses one of the most profuse blood supplies in the body. In growing bone, however, there are areas in which injury and disease can readily imperil the nutrition to vital cellular functions. The diaphysis and metaphysis are provided with nutrition by both extramedullary periosteal vessels and intramedullary vessels that arise from the long vessels in the limb and course through the muscle and fibrous channels to gain access to bone. The penetrating intramedullary vessel primarily supplies the endosteum in the metaphyseal regions.

The epiphyseal and physeal regions obtain nutrition by a potentially more precarious route. The epiphysis is fed by branches that run subperiosteally in the metaphysis, cross the perichondrial ring, and penetrate the perichondrium just above the germinal-resting zone of the growth plate (Figure 1.3). These vessels then run on the physeal side of the epiphyseal ossification center and then arborize into the epiphyseal ossification center. These vessels supply the epiphyseal ossification center as well as a portion of the subchondral side of the intra-articular cartilage. The articular surface cartilage of the epiphysis is believed to derive the majority of its nutrition primarily from the synovium of the joint by a process of direct diffusion. The vessels that supply the epiphyseal ossification center also provide the sole source of nutrition for the germinal and proliferative zones of the growth plate by diffusion of nutrients. Unfortunately, injury or disease that impairs the delicate vascularity to the epiphyseal ossification center will also likely damage the critical growing cells

Figure 1.3. The vascular supply to the secondary ossification center and physis in a child with an established growth plate.

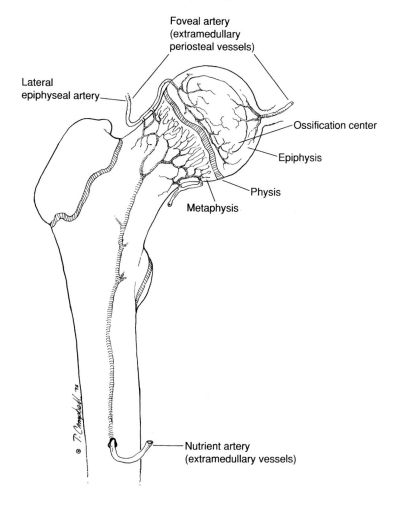

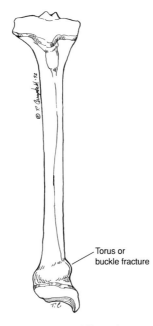

Figure 1.4. A torus or buckle fracture seen commonly as a "toddler's" fracture of the tibia in young children.

of the growth plate with ensuing damage to future longitudinal growth.

Responses to stress

The peculiar anatomy and physiology of growing bone compared with adult bone influence its ability to respond to stresses, whether they are traumatic in origin or internally destructive (such as infection or tumor). The abundance of immature cancellous bone in the metaphysis renders the bone intrinsically fragile and porous in nature thus helping to explain the nature of compression failure (i.e., torus or buckle fractures) (Figure 1.4). Infection may easily penetrate to the weaker, less dense "honeycomb" metaphyseal region as well. The abundance of cartilage at the ends of the long bones affords good shock absorption but provides far less durability in resisting larger forces than the densely compacted adult type of cortical and cancellous bone.

The rich vascularity and abundant cells capable of producing bone seen commonly in the periosteal and endosteum regions allow growing bone to continually remodel, realigning itself along the lines of stress and reconstituting form and shape to ward off the ravages of any offending insult. This remarkable reparative capacity seen throughout our growing years is probably responsible for our successful survival into adulthood.

Contributions to longitudinal growth

The long bones of the extremities and the flat bones of the spine and pelvis vary in the amount of their contribution to our overall height and also vary in relation to the location of growth centers within the given bone. It is known that roughly 60 percent of growth contribution in the spine is achieved by four years of age, and by skeletal age 10 years it is likely that 80 percent of all spinal growth has been achieved. By 10 years of skeletal age, roughly 80 percent of all foot growth has already occurred and 90 percent is completed by skeletal age of 13 years.

The amount and location of growth within a given bone is genetically governed, and further controlled in concert with hormonal input as well as the overall state of nutrition. As an example, marked changes in height during puberty reflect our genetic predestination coupled with the delicate balance and mix of the hormones of puberty (growth hormone, thyroid hormone, and sex hormones). This major "burst" in height predominantly occurs at the level of our knees, where contributions from the distal femoral and proximal tibial epiphyses account for over 70 percent of the entire length of the lower limbs (Figure 1.5).

The relative differences in growth contributions by the physes at either end of the long bones mirror the variations in the blood supply and the level of metabolic activity at a given site. The distal femoral growth plate contributes much more to overall femoral length and overall limb length than the proximal femoral growth plate, which contributes only 11 to 12 percent of the entire length of the limb (Figure 1.6). The proximal tibial and fibular growth plates contribute significantly more than the distal tibial and fibular growth plates both to the length of the tibial and fibular segments and to the overall length of the limb.

There is a role reversal in the upper extremity, where the proximal humeral growth plate is much more metabolically active than the distal humeral. Likewise, the distal radial and ulnar epiphyses contribute far more to the overall length of the upper extremity than does the proximal radius and ulna. This unique arrangement of varying contributions to growth reflects differing levels of metabolic activity and provides a likely explanation for the greater incidence of infections, tumors, and growth disorders occurring in the areas of greatest metabolic activity and in the areas of greatest contribution to longitudinal growth.

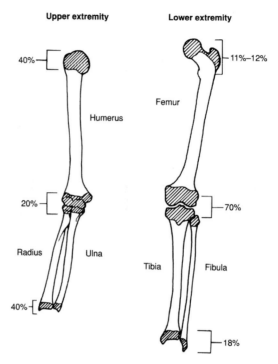

Figure 1.5. The percentage of contribution of growth to the entire extremity.

Figure 1.6. The percentage of growth contribution provided by the growth plates of the bones within the extremity.

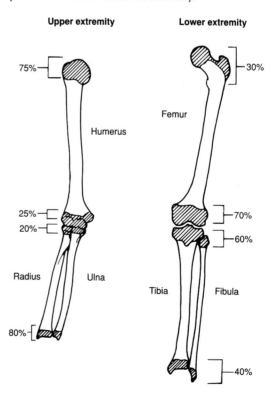

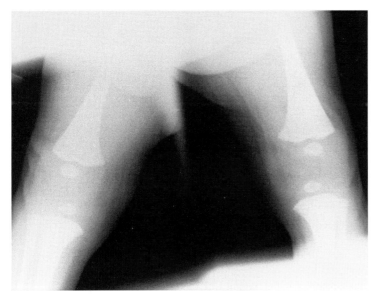

Figure 1.7. Neonatal radiograph showing ossification of the distal femoral and proximal tibial epiphyses at birth.

Skeletal maturation concepts

From birth to skeletal maturity the end of the long bones and growth centers evolve in a predictable fashion, providing height and width to our skeleton. The ends of the long bones become converted from cartilage into bone, eventually covered by a thin layer of articular (joint) cartilage. The growth plate cartilage thins with age, and eventually disappears after fulfilling its mission. The diaphysis converts into a cylindrical form with dense hard osteonal bone remarkably adapted to withstand stress (particularly in compression, and relatively well in rotation and bending).

At birth the distal femoral epiphysis is usually ossified, as is the proximal tibial epiphysis (Figure 1.7). The proximal femoral epiphysis generally does not ossify until three to six months of age. The shoulder and elbow epiphyses and the distal radius and ulnar epiphyses are not ossified at birth. The talus, calcaneus, and the cuboid are partially ossified at birth. Skeletal maturation in the female generally occurs, on average, at a rate of one and a half years ahead of the male. This skeletal growth disparity persists throughout puberty until the cessation of skeletal growth.

Skeletal age determinations, which are much more accurate than chronological age determinations, are also subject to many variables but provide a useful guide in most pathologic states. Skeletal age determination prior to adolescence (i.e., age five, six, and seven years) is usually done by assessing the extent of the appearance of epiphyseal ossification centers. This technique is much less accurate than skeletal age determination in teenagers. In the adolescent/ puberty group, bone ages are generally believed to be accurate to within plus or minus six months, and are performed by comparing radiographs, particularly in regards to the degree of maturation and fusion of the epiphyses (Figure 1.8). Most commonly the hand is utilized for comparison but some believe

Table 1.1 *Height multiplier by age for boys and girls*

Age (years)	Boys	Girls
0	3.14	3.00
1	2.37	2.28
2	2.08	1.97
3	1.89	1.79
4	1.74	1.65
5	1.63	1.54
6	1.54	1.45
7	1.46	1.37
8	1.39	1.31
9	1.33	1.25
10	1.28	1.20
11	1.23	1.15
12	1.19	1.09
13	1.15	1.05
14	1.10	1.03
15	1.05	1.02
16	1.02	1.00
17	1.01	1.00
18	1.00	1.00

Paley, D. (2002). *Principles of Deformity Correction*, pp. 697–715. Berlin: Springer-Verlag. (Chart supplied in envelope in back of book.)

additional accuracy can be obtained using the maturation of the distal femoral and proximal tibial physes. The iliac crest will also begin to ossify originally from its anterolateral extremity, and over a 12- to 18-month period progressively ossify and transit to its posterior medial extension, at which time the apophysis is described as demonstrating *capping*. It has been generally accepted that very little, if any spinal growth in length will occur when capping occurs. Fusion of the epiphyses connotes true maturation, but in many areas this occurs much later than longitudinal growth cessation. Skeletal maturation in females tends to occur at the average of 15 to 15.5 years, while skeletal maturation in the male generally occurs later at 16.5 to 17 years. In 2000, Paley developed a method for predicting the adult height of children of various ages. This "multiplier" method is currently the most accurate formula available (Table 1.1).

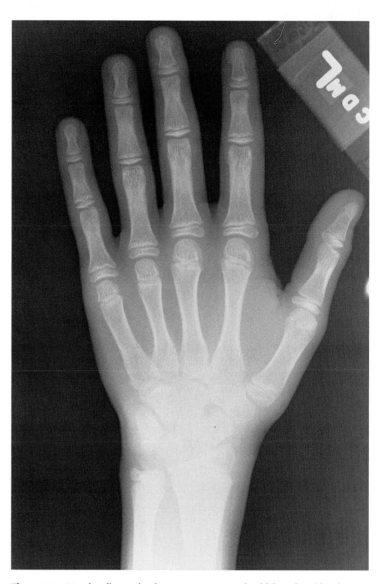

Figure 1.8. Hand radiograph of a 13-year 11-month-old female with a bone age (skeletal age) of 12 years.

Chapter 2

Lower extremity developmental attitudes in infancy and early childhood

If we cannot alter the natural history of a condition, then it is perhaps wise to spare the patient the consequences of our attempts.

I. Macnab, personal communication.

Normal attitudes of the lower extremities (birth to 18 months)

It is surprising how common it is for parents to seek medical attention for "apparent" deformities of the lower extremities from birth to 18 months of age. Undoubtedly, as physicians, we have done a less than adequate job in educating parents as to the "normal" lower extremity attitudes in young children.

At birth, following a cephalic or breech delivery, the hips will characteristically lie in flexion with a flexion contracture commonly of 30–60 degrees (Figure 2.1). Likewise, a knee flexion contracture of 20–45 degrees is not at all uncommon, except following a frank breech delivery. There are usually 10–30 degrees of internal tibial torsion, and the position of the foot and ankle will be a direct reflection of intrauterine posturing. Consequently, equinovarus, equinovalgus, calcaneovalgus, and calcaneovarus are all normal accompaniments providing that the deformity is fully flexible and passively correctable beyond the neutral position. Intrauterine postural deformities secondary to normal intrauterine compression will generally unwind and spontaneously correct, usually by three months of age, in well over 90 percent of all children. Treatment of these deformities by

Figure 2.1. The degree of knee and hip joint contracture commonly seen at birth.

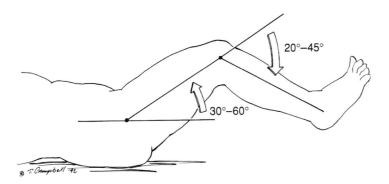

20°–45°

30°–60°

© T. Campbell '92

parental positioning, stretching, splints, casts, or braces will be universally successful, with little more scientific merit than having the parents pay periodic visits to the zoo until the child is four months of age.

Although hip contracture generally spontaneously improves, a mild contracture of 15–20 degrees is common even at six to nine months of age, until the child begins standing through much of his or her waking day. Likewise, the knee contracture will unwind, although full straightening is uncommon until standing is achieved. Internal tibial torsion also will spontaneously improve (this process will be covered in a later discussion). Intrauterine foot and ankle deformation has an identical evolution, with flexibility increasing rapidly through the first three months of extrauterine life. The 10–15 percent of children who persist beyond that age with contracture will be dealt with subsequently. It is conceptually easy to envision the rationale for these postural attitudes. There is little necessity for "straight" hips, knees, ankles, and feet in a child who is rolling over, sitting, and crawling. When "mother nature" determines that it is time to stand and eventually walk, the bones and joints will then allow for that attitude without our interference.

Out-toeing

Nearly 90 percent of all adults who have been clinically measured will have zero to ten degrees of out-toeing as a part of their normal gait pattern. So common is this complaint seen by primary care physicians and pediatric orthopedists, that I have devoted a separate discussion to the topic. At birth, nearly all children have 70–90 degrees of passive and active external rotation of the hip, regardless of the degree of hip flexion contracture. The normal crowded intrauterine position does not allow the infant to "stand up," or to internally rotate the lower limbs. Consequently, external

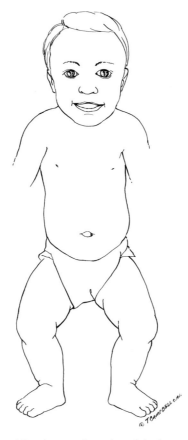

Figure 2.2. Normal early stance. "Crouch" and external rotation of the lower extremities and foot pronation.

rotation at the hip level is the "norm" and this contracture deformation persists until it is no longer needed. There is little need for internal rotation of the hip until children begin to crawl and particularly until they begin to stand. Lower limbs that are externally rotated and abducted are helpful for initially achieving appropriate standing balance and stability.

Considering the needs that our body has for the age that we are, it is amazing that we are "lined up and ready to go" when we achieve that next developmental milestone. Just as a mechanical engineer would design a modern sports car for stability and balance by lowering the center of gravity and widening its base, so do we humans spread our legs (widen the base), externally rotate our hips, crouch or squat (lower our center of gravity), and even pronate or "inroll" our ankles to achieve a maximally stable weight bearing surface for our feet (Figure 2.2). Nearly every grandmother will recognise this posture, as all of her "normal" grandchildren will have demonstrated it when they began to stand and walk.

Physicians need only assure themselves and the parents that the hips are well located, and that no other hip deformity exists. *Developmental* displacement of the hips (formerly termed congenital dislocation of the hip), congenital coxa vara, partial absence of the femur, and neurologic disorders of the lower extremity are uncommon causes of external rotation that should be considered. However, a properly conducted history and physical, and perhaps a radiograph if clearly clinically indicated, will establish the benign nature of the observation. In addition to the expense of unnecessary braces, splints, and adaptive shoe wear to treat this condition, there is a psychological impact of implanting within families' minds the idea that their "loved one" is "diseased," and this should provide adequate caution to all of us. There is nothing medically demeaning in simply reassuring the family, particularly when the consequences of treatment will only perpetuate the fallacy.

Genu varum ("bowlegs") and genu valgum ("knock-knees")

From the 1940s to the present, "bowlegs" and "knock-knees" have enjoyed the distinction of being one of the most common complaints seen by primary care physicians and orthopedic surgeons. A far greater understanding of the natural evolution of these conditions in childhood has resulted in a dramatic reduction in the number of these cases currently seen by physicians.

In addressing the natural history of these two conditions in the growing child, it is important to exclude those cases associated with nutritional or vitamin D resistant rickets, Blount's disease, skeletal chondro-osseous dysplasia, traumatic growth plate insults, infection, and neoplasm. If there is any question, a careful history coupled with radiographs taken of the knees and occasionally laboratory tests are capable of differentiating these conditions from the physiologic type of varus and valgus that will be discussed. Over the past 20 years, several articles have clearly shown that the natural history of physiologic varus and valgus follows a clear and defined pathway (Figure 2.3). From birth to roughly 18 months of age, there is a normal "varoid" stage of development in which bowed legs persist. From 24 months onward, children normally will enter a stage of increasing valgus at the knees and this generally will persist until adolescence, at which time they seem to follow a pattern of their genetic inheritance, eventually culminating into a pattern of knees that are either straight or with very minor degrees of varus or valgus. Varus and valgus at knee level is most readily measured by placing the ankles together at the medial malleoli, and measuring the number of "fingerbreadths" that can be placed between the medial femoral condyles (bowed legs or varus) (Figure 2.4). Knock-knee or valgus deformity is most readily measured by bringing the medial femoral condyles together and then measuring the distance

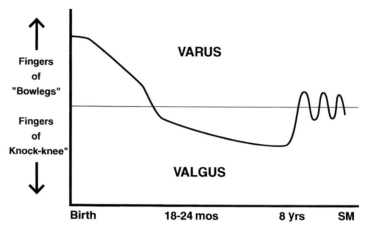

Figure 2.3. Graph demonstrating physiologic progression of varus to valgus. SM: Skeletal Maturity.

Figure 2.4. The technique of measurement by finger-breadths of genu varum and genu valgum.

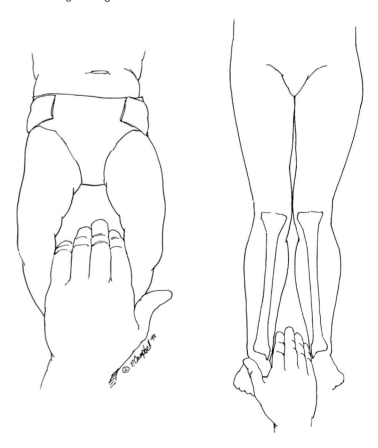

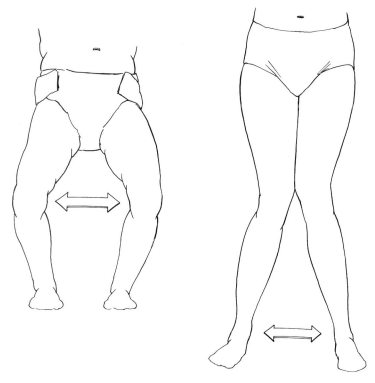

Figure 2.5. The technique of measurement by centimeters or inches of genu varum and genu valgum.

Pearl 2.1. Differential diagnosis of physiologic genu varum

Blount's disease
Skeletal dysplasias
Nutritional rickets
Vit D resistant rickets
Growth plate insult
Infection
Neoplasm

---

between the medial malleoli with the knees in the extended position. A simple recording of the number of fingers measured on each visit will provide irrefutable evidence of the natural evolution of the angular deviation. It has also been commonly observed that youngsters who walk early (i.e., at 9–10 months of age) will commonly have more genu varum, which will tend to persist even into the second and early third year of life before spontaneous resolution into valgus occurs. An alternative method of following the process clinically is to make drawings on a sheet of paper of the contour of the knees in relationship to the ankles, and then measuring the distance between the various anatomic landmarks on a sheet of paper (Figure 2.5).

Historically these physiologic angular alterations have been treated by stretching, shoe adaptations, orthotics, medications, surgical epiphyseal stapling, and osteotomy of the long bones. In the absence of a known medical disease or disorder (Pearl 2.1), physiologic genu varum and genu valgum will spontaneously resolve into an acceptable degree of knee alignment by maturity. Our own extensive experience has failed to provide any cases presenting for treatment at skeletal maturity. Periodic follow-up and reassurance to ameliorate parental anxiety appears to be all that is necessary.

Metatarsus adductus

Metatarsus adductus is the least common cause of in-toeing seen in infants and children. It has occasionally been termed "monkey-toeing" due to the peculiar deviation of the great toe medially resembling that seen in arboreal apes, while the lateral four toes tend to be pointing in a straight position. The condition is most commonly seen from birth to 18 months and may persist until three years of age. It is characterized by a flexible medial deviation of the great toe, not unlike that seen in primates with a prehensile first digit. It is most commonly believed to be due to persistence of activity of the abductor hallucis muscle (Figure 2.6). The natural propensity for metatarsus adductus is to resolve spontaneously, and this casts doubt on the wisdom of using any active treatment. Occasionally adaptive shoes and orthotics have been utilized, but they should be viewed as unnecessary.

Metatarsus adductovarus

Metatarsus adductovarus is nearly as common a cause of in-toeing as internal tibial torsion. It has been known in the past by a number of different terms, all of which seem to create more confusion that reason. It has been referred to as "one-third of a clubfoot," congenital "hooked" forefoot, forefoot adductus, forefoot adductovarus, metatarsus internus, metatarsus varus, and metatarsus "supinatus." The key differentiating feature between metatarsus adductovarus and metatarsus adductus is that in metatarsus adductovarus there is an adduction deformity of the forefoot, coupled with a supination deformity of the forefoot in relationship to a normal hindfoot. Put more simply, it is a "stiff" supination deformity or varus deformity of the forefoot on the hindfoot. It is further characterized by a medial and plantar crease, beginning just distal to the navicular and medial cuneiform region, and extending roughly halfway across the plantar aspect of the foot (Figures 2.7 & 2.8).

The etiology of this condition is unknown, but it is believed to occur antenatally and is likely related to intrauterine factors, particularly inadequate intrauterine space. It is commonly classified as a form of intrauterine "molding." Not unlike developmental dislocation of the hip, the natural history of this condition is reflected in the fact that roughly 85 percent of all feet so affected will spontaneously resolve without any significant treatment being given. This finding lends

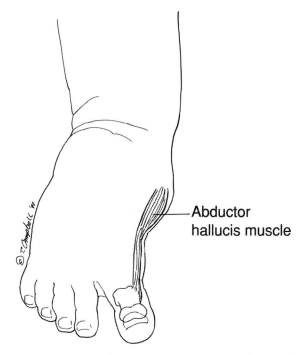

Abductor hallucis muscle

Figure 2.6. The activity of the abductor hallucis muscle tendon unit in producing metatarsus adductus.

Figure 2.7. The typical clinical deformity in metatarsus adductovarus, including the deep medial and plantar crease.

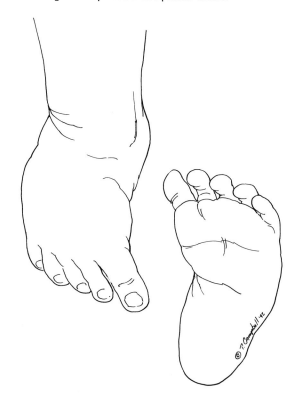

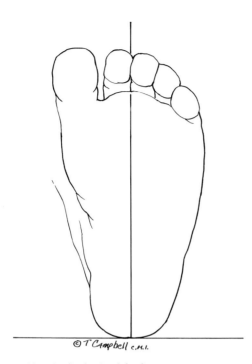

Figure 2.8. Drawing of normal longitudinal axis of the foot.

Figure 2.9. The position of the hands in relationship to the foot in testing the degree of flexibility of metatarsus adductovarus.

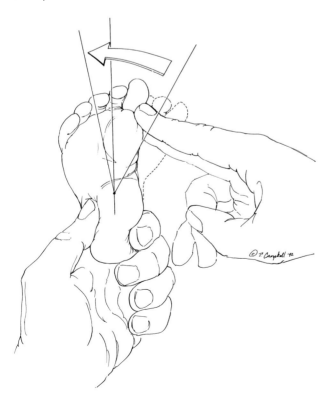

credence to the suggestion that intrauterine molding factors play a major part in etiology.

Normally, gentle two-finger pressure across the forefoot, while holding the hindfoot in a stable position, will easily overcorrect the "deformity" in the type of metatarsus adductovarus that will spontaneously resolve (Figure 2.9). In children who have not resolved the deformity by three months of age, and in whom it is not possible to reverse the position of the forefoot on the hindfoot beyond the normal longitudinal axis of the foot, treatment is usually instituted. A wide variety of treatment modalities have been utilized, consisting primarily of adaptive shoe wear alone, or in combination with various orthotics. Serial plaster casting is also one of the most common forms of treatment used. Success in treating this condition has routinely been obtained by the use of serial casting, bar and shoes in combination, and shoe-brace combination devices designed to create a prono-valgus force across the foot. Less than five percent of all patients will persist with residual deformity of sufficient cosmetically deforming nature to require surgical correction.

The residuals of this condition result in a cosmetic deformity that has never been shown to be functionally impairing. However, occasionally the forefoot deformation is sufficient to interfere with purchasing "over-the-counter" non-prescription shoes, which generates a great deal of parental concern, leading them to pressure for surgical correction.

Internal tibial torsion

Internal tibial torsion constitutes the second most common cause of in-toeing presenting to the physician and the pediatric orthopedist. In contrast to *developmental femoral anteversion*, it presents much earlier, commonly seen initially between three months and two years of age. Nearly as many cases present for diagnosis and treatment prior to walking age as ever appear thereafter. The condition is manifest in both sexes equally.

The child presents to the physician initially with limbs that are "inturned." The "deformity" is evident during gait, or even in the supine position, or sitting with the legs over the side of the table with the knee in the flexed position. There is an inward medial rotation of the ankle and foot relative to the proximal (tibial and fibular) position of the leg. On examination, the maximum prominence of the tibial tubercle is discerned, and the maximal prominence of the medial and lateral malleoli is determined. The degree of internal tibial torsion is measured as the degree of clinical rotation inwards of the "dorsiflexed" foot as it relates to the tibial tubercle (Figures 2.10 & 2.11). Other techniques of measurement include radiographs and the use of specialized calipers. Unfortunately, all methods fall prey to inherent variability in positioning of the parts to be examined, the selection of distinct and reproducible anatomic landmarks, and the incomplete and irregular ossification of the tibia and fibula seen in the age group presenting for examination. It is to be emphasized that this condition is a "clinical diagnosis."

Being a result of intrauterine positioning, internal tibial torsion is likely a common physiologic feature of almost all neonates and in most normal youngsters in the first year of life. The natural benign evolution of this condition is undoubtedly the single most important piece of information to be retained. It is virtually never encountered in adolescents and teenagers unless associated with pathologic conditions. The large numbers of very young children seen with this condition, and the near total absence of teenagers, suggest that spontaneous recovery routinely occurs. There is substantial clinical scientific evidence to support the fact that spontaneous resolution occurs, and likely occurs as a compensation both through the ankle and foot, and probably through the hip and knee as well.

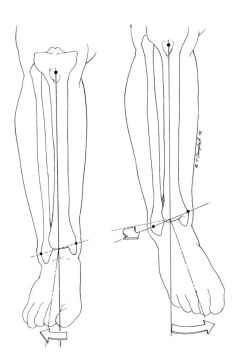

Figure 2.10. The relationship of the medial and lateral malleolus relative to the center of the tibial tubercle in both the normal state and in the presence of internal tibial torsion.

Figure 2.11. Drawing of internal tibial torsion as viewed from proximal to distal tibia.

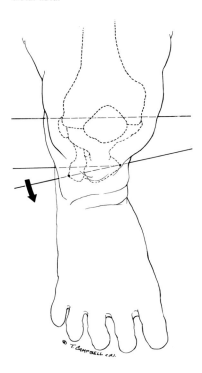

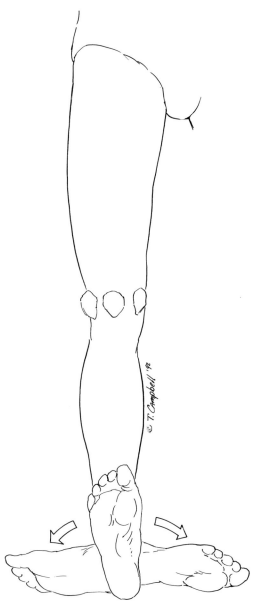

Figure 2.12. The large degree of hip rotation possible in normal children. A considerable range of internal rotation is routinely present in the clinical condition of developmental femoral anteversion (hip in-toeing).

Treatment, which has consisted of altering sleeping and sitting positions, a wide assortment of braces and shoe/brace combinations, "twister" cables, serial casting, and even surgical derotation osteotomy must be considered superfluous in light of our current knowledge of natural history.

Developmental femoral anteversion ("hip in-toeing")

The most common cause of in-toeing seen in children is developmental femoral anteversion, or more appropriately, "hip in-toeing." The physician will not likely pass through a week of clinical practice without seeing a patient with this complaint. Patients are generally brought to the examining physician by the parents who are concerned that the child "toes in" during gait, walks "pigeon toed", or is constantly tripping or stumbling. Most commonly, the symptoms are magnified by running, tiredness, or commonly encountered when the patient is not fully conscious of the in-toeing. The maximum incidence of presentation is between two and eight years of age. Both sexes are affected equally and the clinical findings essentially mirror the symptomatology.

On examination, the hips characteristically will have a great deal of internal rotation, both with the hips extended and flexed, commonly approaching 90 degrees (Figure 2.12). External rotation in both flexion and extension of the hip may range from 15–20 degrees, all the way up to 90 degrees of external rotation. Providing the child is in no way neurologically handicapped or has a fixed contracture of the hip joint, there is no evidence to suggest that the degree of internal rotation will vary in either the flexed or extended position of the hip.

In all probability, the increased range of motion of the hip is a function of the very young child, whose joint ranges of motion, in general, far exceed that which will be present at the time of skeletal maturity. Laymen have always been aware that we become "stiffer" in our joints with age and it is clearly supported in the decreasing range of hip motion normally seen from birth to puberty. Inasmuch as the child has a very wide range of motion, particularly in internal rotation, it is quite comfortable for them to sit in a "W" position or a reverse "tailor" position (Figure 2.13). It is also more comfortable for them to walk internally rotated during gait, particularly when they are tired or running. Personal experience, using computed tomography scanning, does *not* support any increase in the bending of the upper end of the bony femur in relationship to the acetabulum (anteversion), an anatomic event erroneously attributed to the etiology. It is paradoxical that at birth, when true bony anteversion is at the greatest degree in the human, the range of external rotation of the hip is the greatest, as it will be throughout the first year of life. Furthermore, internal rotation of the hip and subsequent hip in-toeing, seen as a clinically manifested condition, occurs most commonly between two and eight years of age, at a time in development when anatomic bony anteversion is beginning to spontaneously diminish (Figure 2.14).

A wide variety of treatment modalities have been used in managing this condition, ranging from alterations in sitting and sleeping positions, adaptive-corrective shoe wear, and a myriad of braces (orthotics). Even surgical derotation osteotomies have been recommended in a few selected cases if spontaneous correction fails. There is, however, no scientific evidence to support that any treatment, in any way, affects the ultimate outcome of this condition. In fact, there is substantial supporting information that the natural history of this condition is to resolve spontaneously by the attainment of skeletal maturation. The exact mechanics of how this resolution occurs is as yet obscure, although it is well known that there is definitely a reduction in the degree of range of motion of the hips as one matures. Additionally, there is ample

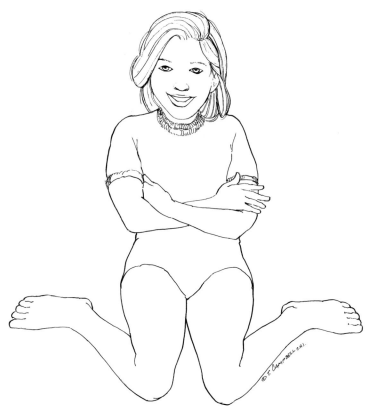

Figure 2.13. Characteristic "W" sitting position assumed in children with hip in-toeing.

Figure 2.14. Normal recession of femoral anteversion (in degrees) with growth.

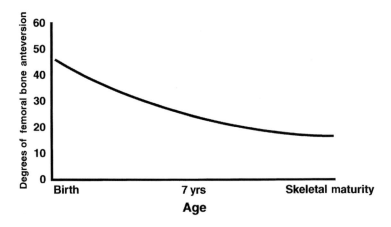

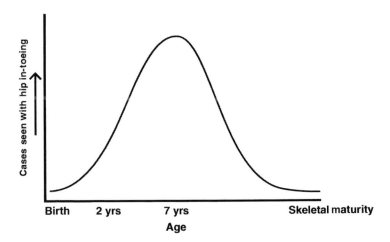

Figure 2.15. Distribution by age of clinical cases of hip in-toeing.

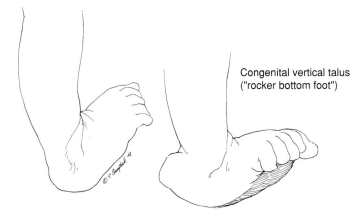

Figure 2.16. The differences in clinical appearance between flexible calcaneovalgus and congenital vertical talus.

Flexible calcaneovalgus

Congenital vertical talus ("rocker bottom foot")

evidence to support the fact that external tibial rotation naturally develops in normal children as they progress through the adolescent age group. Patients examined, prospectively, clearly show a marked increase in the development of external tibial rotation in the face of substantial internal femoral rotation.

Regardless of the mechanism of resolution, it is virtually impossible to find a suitable candidate who has achieved skeletal maturity, who is substantially disabled (i.e., in-turning) to allow themselves to submit to surgical derotation osteotomy (Figure 2.15). Treatment of this condition, therefore, should be a matter of parental education and support, as well as physician education as to the natural history of hip in-toeing. Treatment of this condition by any technique must be considered uniformly successful and uniformly unnecessary.

Flexible calcaneovalgus feet

The orthopedic literature prior to 1980 is inundated with a myriad of techniques designed to treat calcaneovalgus deformity of the foot. At one time it was a common misconception to consider it as a type of clubfoot. Because there is little room in the uterus, there are relatively few locations for the foot and ankle to rest. Commonly the ankle and foot are forced into calcaneus, either varus or valgus, and the foot, although moveable and moderately flexible after birth, may persist with a contracture of the ankle in dorsiflexion until roughly three months of age. Occasionally the foot may contact the anterior portion of the distal tibia in severe cases. Twenty to thirty percent of all patients will present at ages up to six months with some degree of residual contracture.

The major differential diagnosis concerns itself with the presence of a congenital vertical talus or *congenital rocker bottom foot*. This rigid deformity is composed of a rigidly plantar flexed talus with a "stiff" contracted mid- and forefoot. Although it may look very much like a flexible calcaneovalgus foot, it is distinguished by clear-cut clinical findings. The heel is rigidly fixed in equinus, and the forefoot is rigidly dorsiflexed on the plantar flexed talus, creating the appearance of a "Persian slipper" or rocker bottom deformity (Figure 2.16). Occasionally a low level (L4–L5) myelodysplasia (spina bifida) patient will present with a calcaneovarus or calcaneovalgus deformity resembling this condition. The history and physical examination should readily serve to differentiate the deformity from that of the flexible postural type.

Treatment for the postural calcaneus foot is usually unnecessary, but sufficient parental concern in those presenting after three months of age may engender the need for attention. Passive stretching exercises prescribed at the time of diaper changes may help allay parental anxiety. Orthotics and adaptive shoe wear are costly, imprudent, and unnecessary.

Congenital curly toes

Although little or no mention of curved deviations of the toes exist in most of our literature and orthopedic textbooks; they are probably one of the most commonly seen "abnormalities" of the foot presenting for treatment. Lateral curving of the second and third toes and inward curving of the fourth and fifth toes account for over 90 percent of these "deformities" and often occur together. Bilaterality is seen in over 75 percent of the cases. The condition is nearly always hereditary. The physical characteristics are an in-or-out curving of the toe, with the apex of angulation between the proximal and distal interphalangeal joints (Figures 2.17a and 2.17b). A contracted skin band on the plantar aspect of the toe is a consistent part of the deformity (Figure 2.18).

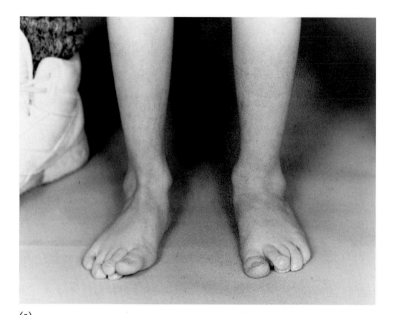

(a)

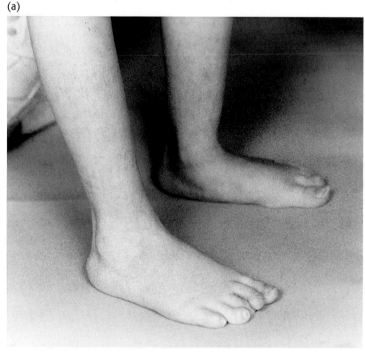

(b)

Figure 2.17. Frontal (a) and lateral (b) views of congenital "curly" toes.

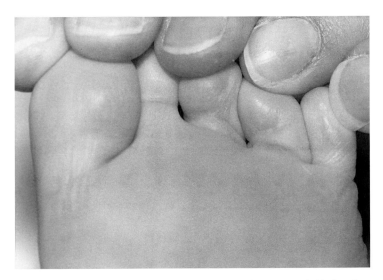

Figure 2.18. Plantar view demonstrating asymmetric contracted skin band seen with "curly" toes.

It is at times difficult to resist temptation to surgically straighten the curly toe, but patience is important. Functional disability (painful corns or calluses) is rarely seen. Furthermore, surgical realignment is often disappointing and may result in substantial scarring, with treatment appearing far worse than the disease.

Chapter 3

Common orthopedic conditions from birth to walking

None will grow more straight in his body than those who are laid free and loose in a sheltered, ample-spaced cradle.

A. V. Neal

Developmental displacement of the hip

The term developmental displacement of the hip has replaced the previous more confining and incriminatory terminology *congenital dislocation of the hip*. Although the vast majority of idiopathic hip dislocations are recognizable at birth, a number of hips will not have sufficient clinical findings of displacement until later in the first year of life (at three to nine months). The implications of this terminology are obvious and the broader spectrum should help clarify our understanding of the evolution of hip displacement, particularly in those in which spontaneous relocation does not occur.

This condition has its origins of recognition with the ancients; Hippocrates aptly described its existence and its treatment. Current concepts of etiology focus primarily on intrauterine and extrauterine factors. Females, first-born children (pressure from strong maternal abdominal muscles), breech malposition and delivery, large body size, oligohydramnios, and genetics have all been strongly implicated as risk factors. This condition is associated with congenital muscular torticollis approximately 20 percent of the time. In those regions of the world where hip extension "strapping" and "cradleboards" are utilized on newborns, the incidence of developmental displacement of the hip occurs approximately 40–50 percent of the time. The highest risk is posed by a first-born, 4.5kg (approx. ten pound) female infant delivered by breech extraction to a primiparous mother with a family history of developmental displacement of the hip. Established dislocation *at birth* is nearly always associated with other disorders such as cerebral palsy, myelodysplasia, arthrogryposis and other syndromes.

It is generally believed that undue pressure on the hip, combined with a lax hip joint capsule (i.e., breech) coupled with strong uterine and abdominal musculature, and large baby size, will sufficiently stretch the hip joint supports and make the hip "dislocatable." This "dislocatability" or instability is commonly evident at birth, and determined by a series of hip examination maneuvers requiring only one to two minutes to perform.

The hip is initially examined with the baby supine and the hips flexed to 90 degrees, and with gentle but firm downward pressure on the femurs to fix the potentially moveable pelvis to the examination table. The fingers are positioned to provide for downward pressure on the femurs and to allow for direct vision of the thighs when abduction and adduction movements are attempted. Asymmetry of the thigh creases is readily appreciated in this position, as are differences in the height of the knees (Figure 3.1). The thighs are then gently and slowly parted (abducted with the middle or ring fingers palpating the greater trochanters). In unstable but "reducible" hips a discernible "clunk" will often be discerned in the neonate but commonly may recede to a "click" over the ensuing few months and then eventually disappear. This easily recognizable "clunk" is termed *Ortolani's sign* (Figure 3.2). The later discernible "click" obtained in near full abduction is usually a sign that the acetabular labrum has not firmly attached and stabilized, but is a sign of improved stability. If a true dislocation is evident, abduction will be clearly limited, as the head will not enter into the

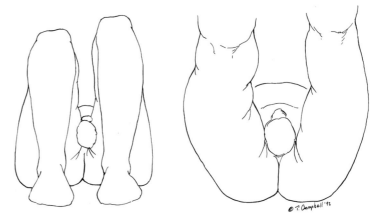

Figure 3.1. The unequal knee heights and asymmetric skin folds in the thigh, seen in developmental displacement of the hip.

Figure 3.2. The technique of eliciting Ortolani's sign.

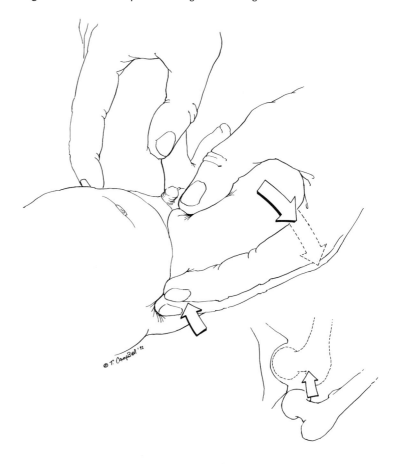

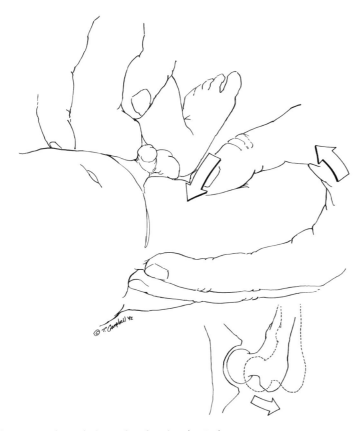

Figure 3.3. The technique of performing the Barlow maneuver.

Figure 3.4. The technique of producing "telescoping" or "pistoning."

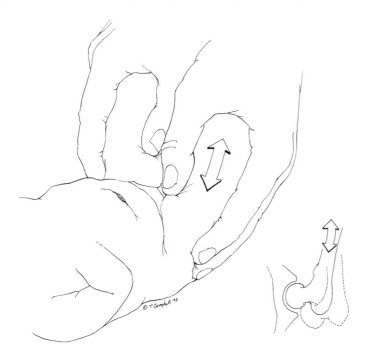

acetabular confines with attempts at reduction. A positive Barlow sign is actually a provocative dislocation or subluxation test, and is elicited using the thumb and fingers to laterally move the femoral head out of the acetabular confines by lateral pressure of the inner aspect of the thigh (Figure 3.3). A discernible "clunk" or "click" will be readily appreciated. Perhaps the most valuable sign of hip instability (subluxation or dislocation) is the "pistoning" or "telescoping" sign. It is generally elicited by stabilizing the pelvis with one hand firmly against the anterior iliac spine, grasping the femur in the other hand, then "pumping" downward and upward in a vertical direction with the hip flexed to 90 degrees (Figure 3.4). The femur will glide up and down within the soft tissue envelope of the thigh and independent of the stable pelvis. As the femur glides within the soft tissue envelope, the pelvis remains fixed with each up and down thrust. A positive "telescoping" sign always reflects hip joint instability. It is imperative that the novice clinically examines as many hips as possible during residency training, as there can never be too many opportunities. The skills achieved in examination are the product of many clinical examinations of both normal and abnormal hips. As the child approaches six months of age, dislocation may lead to an adduction contracture, and reduction of the hip becomes much more difficult with the disappearance of the Ortolani sign. Diagnosis in the ambulatory child should be much easier with shortening, limp, and telescoping more obvious.

The natural history or evolution of a displaced hip in infancy has been the topic of considerable investigation and commentary. Most people agree that there is a tremendous tendency for the hip to stabilize spontaneously, with a likelihood of 85–90 percent of all hips achieving stabilization by 9–10 months of age. Unfortunately, we are presently unable to predict which hips will stabilize, and we are left with 10–15 percent who will remain with varying degrees of hip malpositioning, including even frank dislocation. The future of hip joint function appears directly related to the early recognition of this problem. Careful hip examination should take place from birth to one year of age at regular intervals.

The role of radiographic examination or the use of ultrasound is less clearly defined. The femoral head does not normally ossify its secondary ossification center until roughly three to six months of age, and that ossification of the center is commonly delayed even further in developmental displacement of the hip. While there is nothing wrong with performing an imaging examination at three to six months of age, particularly in high risk infants, it should never replace a careful hip examination. Bilaterally involved hips pose the greater hazard, and make the individual hip examination even more important, as "widening" of the perineum seen in bilaterality is very difficult to discern in infants and young children.

Radiographic examination of the hips in very young children is fraught with potential misinterpretation errors. To be at all meaningful, anteroposterior examination must be done with the hips and knees maximally extended, and with the patella directed vertically (Figure 3.5). Abduction views of the hips tend to induce femoral head relocation, and external rotation positioning promotes lateralization of an already anteverted femoral head and neck. At birth nearly 40 percent of the acetabulum is formed in cartilage. If one couples that information with the fact that the femoral head is for all parts a chondroepiphysis, with an occasional degree of secondary ossification, it is possible to visualize only a small portion of the hip joint on plain radiography in the very young child (Figures 3.6a, b and 3.7a, b).

Currently the use of ultrasound has gained an increasingly important role in the diagnosis and even the management of developmental dislocation of the hip. Ultrasound in the hands of a competent examiner can provide useful information regarding the femoral head and acetabular relationship particularly prior to the

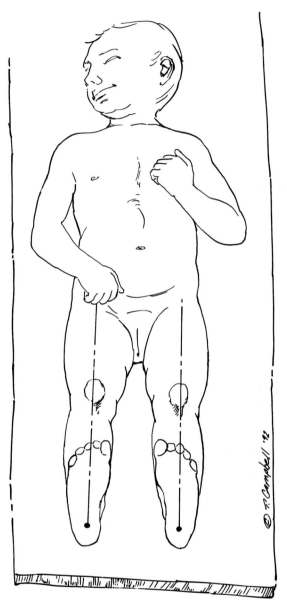

Figure 3.5. The positioning of the child for standard anteroposterior radiographs of the hip.

(a)

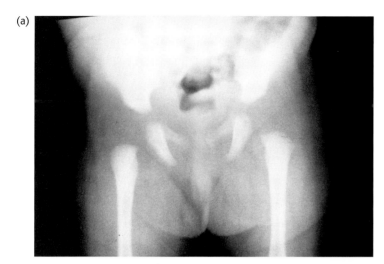

(b)

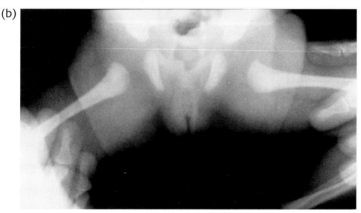

Figure 3.6. Anteroposterior (a) and lateral (b) radiographs of neonate highlighting the absence of the ossification center and the large amount of femoral head/acetabulum that is not visible on standard radiographs at this age.

appearance of the secondary center of ossification of the femoral head. It is to be emphasized that the individual performing the ultrasound test be very experienced as the provocative testing is extremely critical and the learning curve can be steep.

In the first month of life, many children who in fact do not have developmental dislocation of the hip, will have sufficient normal "laxity" of the soft tissue that provide hip joint stability to produce false-positive instability on ultrasound that will spontaneously disappear on later testing. Given this normal sequence of events, ultrasound is probably best utilized between one month of age and prior to the appearance of the ossified femoral head. It is merely an additional imaging technique to assist the primary care physician's arsenal of evaluation techniques.

Ultrasound is safe, noninvasive and does not involve the use of ionizing radiation although it is currently much more expensive than conventional radiography. In the presence of risk factors for developmental dislocation of the hip, it would seem appropriate to screen patients with ultrasound when they are four to six weeks of age. The number of risk factors that need to be present to initiate the ultrasound testing is still very controversial. *None* of the currently available "imaging" techniques should replace a careful clinical examination.

Once a displaced hip is recognized at birth or shortly after birth, the hip should be allowed to lie in the fetal human position of flexion and unforced abduction. Nearly 50 percent of all "displaced" femoral heads will relocate in the first 30–45 days of life, and a simple soft device that provides flexion above 90 degrees and abduction of roughly 45–60 degrees is usually adequate (double/triple diapers, pillow splints, abduction brace or harness). If signs of clinical hip instability persist beyond this point, a more concerted effort to contain the hip is generally indicated (rigid splint, Ilfeld type brace, Pavlik harness, hip abduction cast). Treatment is generally employed for six weeks to three months for unstable, but not dislocated hips. Frank hip dislocation in children three months to one year of age are generally best treated by manual relocation under anesthesia often combined with adductor tenotomy if necessary, a hip spica cast, or by brace or harness reduction. The length of treatment time is usually three to six months. Failures of this treatment regime will likely require surgical repositioning, and often femoral and pelvic realignment procedures to maintain hip stability.

Clearly the overall role of the primary care physician rests with the diagnosis, where early or late recognition likely will determine the ultimate prognosis for future hip stability. However, some few cases will escape detection, even in the hands of competent examiners, and be recognized only later (at nine to ten months of age) when the clinical signs can be more readily perceived (Figure 3.8).

Congenital idiopathic clubfoot

The term *talipes equinovarus* is derived from the Latin word *talipes* (talus:ankle; pes:foot) and *equinus* (horse-like), and *varus* (inverted or adducted), and is exquisitely descriptive of the deformity. It is estimated to occur in roughly one of every 1000 live births. It occurs more commonly in males, and occurs bilaterally in nearly 50 percent of all cases. If a first-born male is affected, there is nearly a 40 times increased incidence of another male being affected. If a second male child is affected, there is nearly a 400 times increase in incidence.

At birth the deformity is readily recognized, although some feet are more rigid than others. It is the feature of rigidity that separates the deformity from postural intrauterine positioning. The components of rigidity are a forefoot adduction and supination, termed *adductovarus*, combined with inversion or supination of the hindfoot (varus) and equinus of the hindfoot (fixed plantar flexion)

(a)

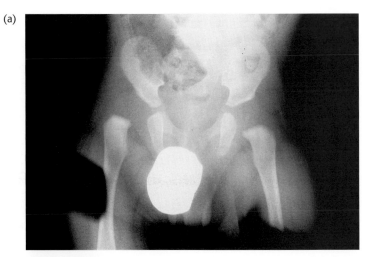

(b)

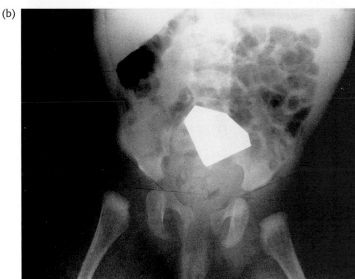

Figure 3.7. Anteroposterior (a) and lateral (b) radiographs demonstrating hip subluxation in a young child prior to ossification of the secondary center of the femoral head.

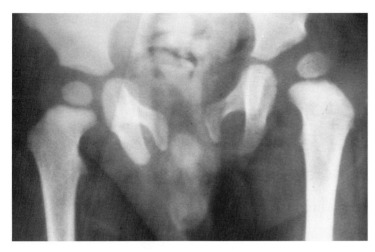

Figure 3.8. Anteroposterior radiograph of an 8-month-old child with a "late appearing" developmental displacement of the hip.

Figure 3.9. Frontal (a) and lateral (b) views of idiopathic rigid clubfoot.

(a)

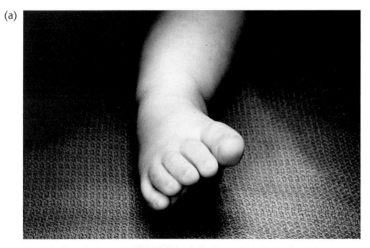

(b)

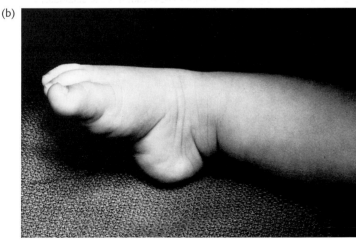

(Figures 3.9a, b). Even with manipulation, the foot cannot be reduced into a normal position.

At the present time the exact etiology is obscure, but there are several theories, none fully substantiated, that are embraced by many orthopedic surgeons. One group believes that the clubfoot is a germ plasm defect, in which the talus never develops into a normal size and shape, and that all other deformities seen are secondary to the primary talar deformity. The second school of thought centers on the clubfoot being a neuromuscular disorder, not previously described, which results in all observed deformities occurring as sequelae of neuromuscular imbalance. Some believe clubfeet are a regional form of arthrogryposis. The talar deformity is viewed as a secondary phenomenon. Regardless of which of the theories is eventually proven correct, it is clear that the talus is always deformed, with a foreshortened talar neck that is always medially and plantar deviated. This typical deformity of the talus has been visualized in nearly all stillborn cases who have clubfeet, and in all operative cases to some degree. The navicular also is medially and plantar deflected. The joint capsules on the posteromedial portion of the foot are contracted. The tendons on the posteromedial aspect of the foot (Achilles tendon, flexor hallus longus, flexor digitorium longus, abductor hallucis, posterior tibial tendon, plantar fascia, and short toe flexors) are also contracted. Radiographs are of little value early in life since much of the foot is unossified until much later (at 3–10 years).

There is no medication, stretching program, or orthotic that will overcome the stiffness in a true congenital idiopathic clubfoot. Serial casting followed by orthotic control after correction, or casting combined with surgical releases with or without postoperative orthotics, form the hallmark of treatment. Modern techniques have completely altered the natural history. Left untreated the deformity will insidiously progress. With or without treatment the foot will always be smaller in size and the calf will always be thinner than normal.

The goal of treatment is essentially to achieve a foot that "looks" like a foot, "acts" like a foot, and is a pain-free foot with a substantial weight-bearing surface (plantigrade) (Figures 3.10a, b). Early orthopedic referral to an experienced surgeon will likely result in a near 90 percent chance of obtaining a desirable foot, even if multiple surgeries should become necessary. With early referral and prompt treatment, there is no need for the gloomy outlook routinely encountered in the past.

Congenital muscular torticollis

Congenital muscular torticollis or "wryneck" is a deformity characterized by contracture or contraction of the anterior cervical muscles and fascia, resulting in an abnormal tilting and rotation of the head and neck in relation to the chest. The chin is flexed forward and rotated toward the shoulder opposite from the underlying pathology. Although the term "congenital" persists, it is generally not detected at birth, but appears during the first six weeks of life. It occurs as a consequence of foreshortening of the sternocleidomastoid muscle and fascia. The etiology is unknown although it is commonly associated with breech presentations (30 percent), and developmental displacement of the hip (20 percent). Surgical biopsies have demonstrated changes quite similar to those seen from chronic venous obstruction in muscle, possibly a result of a compartment syndrome. Whether the abnormal contracture precludes normal cephalic delivery, or whether the breech extraction injures the sternocleidomastoid muscle, is still debated. Examination is best conducted with the infant's head extended beyond the edge of the examination table with shoulders stabilized to the table to prevent upper thoracic rotation. The head is then rotated to point the chin to the opposite shoulder (Figure 3.11). Restriction of motion by the tight sternocleidomastoid can be readily palpated. Within the first few weeks

(a)

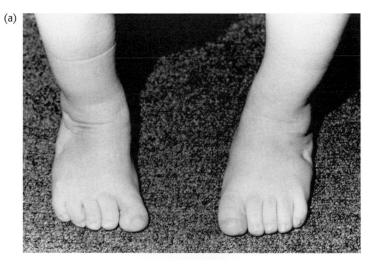

(b)

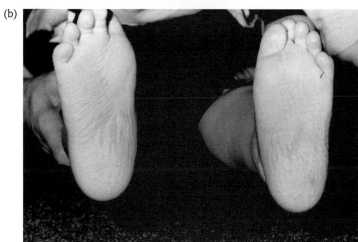

Figure 3.10. (a) Postoperative correction of rigid clubfoot (frontal view). (b) Degree of correction of rigid idiopathic clubfoot (plantar view).

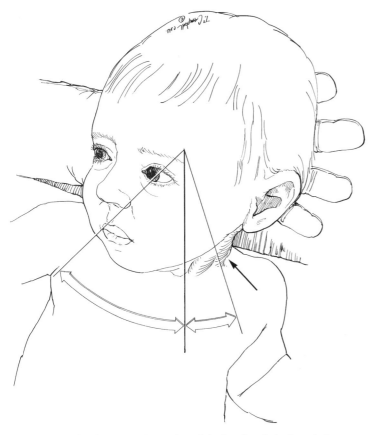

Figure 3.11. The characteristic rotation of the head and plagiocephaly seen in torticollis, and the position for clinical examination.

of life, a semi-firm or firm non-tender mass may be palpable within the substance of the involved sternocleidomastoid. The overlying skin and subcutaneous tissue is freely moveable. The "lump" generally attains its greatest dimension during the first six weeks of life, after which it gradually recedes in size. It will frequently disappear within four to six months, leaving as a residue only the indurated contracted muscle and fascia. Usually the face is flattened and underdeveloped on the ipsilateral side, while the parieto-occipital region on the contralateral side of the skull also flattens (plagiocephaly) (Figure 3.12). The degree of facial and skull deformity is striking and is usually evident at the time of original diagnosis.

The natural history, untreated, is for the condition to slowly progress in the degree of face and head deformity, and in reduced range of motion. Treatment for infants under three months of age consists of stretching (usually repetitive rotations during diaper changes, and turning the bed away from the window to induce the child to rotate toward light). This latter technique is obviously useless when the child is able to roll over. Stretching should persist to 12–18 months of age until correction. Roughly 85 percent of all children will correct by 18 months of age. Beyond 18 months of age, most orthopedic surgeons feel surgical release is the only logical recourse for those who fail conservative care. Surgical release should be performed prior to school age, as craniofacial remodeling diminishes thereafter.

Congenital and infantile scoliosis

Scoliosis from birth to walking age is generally of two types: infantile idiopathic or congenital scoliosis. Infantile idiopathic scoliosis is defined as a spinal curvature making its appearance during the first three years of life. Although it is relatively rare in the United States, it is not uncommon in the UK and Europe. It is more commonly found in males, and shows a preponderance of left-sided thoracic curves (Pearl 3.1). Most of the spinal curvatures are not recognized during the neonatal period but are commonly seen between two and six months of age. In most studies spontaneous improvement or resolution has been observed in well over 50 percent of the patients. The curvatures require close observation, as some of these curves are progressive and can lead to significant deformity. Not uncommonly plagiocephaly, mental retardation, and breech malposition have been associated with a number of the described cases. Because of the difficulty in establishing an appropriate prognosis for these curves, early orthopaedic referral is suggested. Bracing (orthotics) is usually ineffective and surgery is generally reserved for progressive curvatures.

Congenital scoliosis is a result of anomalous vertebral formation (Figure 3.13). Most cases of congenital scoliosis are related either to defects in segmentation of a part, or all, of the vertebrae with resultant fusion of segments, or to failures in formation of a part or all of the vertebrae. Mixed combinations of anomalies in formation are commonly seen. The various types and subtypes of congenital scoliosis are associated with quite different prognostic courses, and the understanding of that evolution more likely should rest in the domain of the orthopedic surgeon. It is, however, important for the primary care physician to be constantly vigilant in the search for other systemic abnormalities in the presence of a congenital scoliosis. The most common associated abnormalities are those involving the bladder, kidneys, heart, and hearing. The embryonic development of these systems occurs in close relationship of the development of the vertebral column. Intraspinal abnormalities such as hydromyelia or diastematomyelia are not uncommonly encountered. Magnetic resonance imaging evaluation should probably be entertained in all cases of congenital scoliosis (vertebral anomalies). In spite of the impressive radiographic nature of many of the cases of

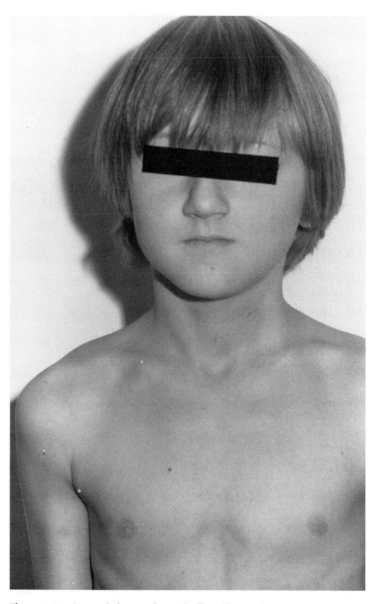

Figure 3.12. Congenital muscular torticollis with prominent sternocleido-mastoid muscle.

Pearl 3.1. Infantile scoliosis

Left thoracic
Males > females
Spontaneous correction
Brace effectiveness

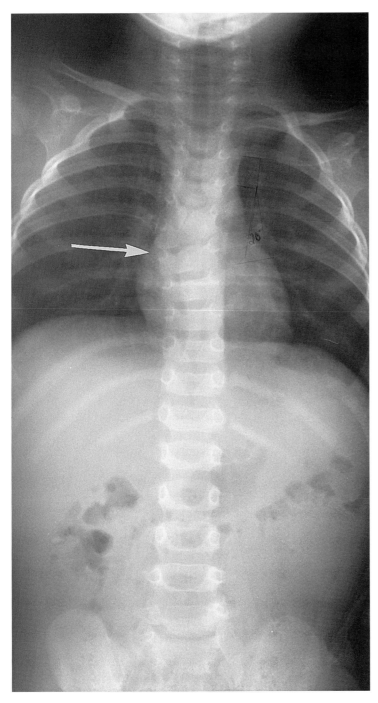

Figure 3.13. Anteroposterior thoracolumbar spine radiograph demonstrating congenital mid-thoracic vertebral anomaly with scoliosis.

congenital scoliosis, not all progress and many are simply observed until maturation. Bracing is rarely, if ever, effective in managing progressive curvatures and surgery is generally the only successful treatment. Early recognition and orthopedic referral are recommended for the primary care physician.

Birth palsies (brachial plexus injuries)

Injuries of the brachial plexus occurring during delivery result in varying degrees of paralysis of the upper extremity. The mechanism of injury is generally a forcible stretching of one or more components of the brachial plexus. Commonly the injuries are a by-product of a difficult delivery involving a large infant. Damage can occur in a cephalic presentation, as a consequence of forced head and neck traction in an effort to deliver broad shoulders through a tight canal. It can also occur in a breech extraction while attempting to deliver the head. Fortunately the nerve roots are rarely completely avulsed, and are usually disrupted with the nerve still in continuity. The degree of severity of the nerve lesion will dictate the rapidity and extent to which the lesion will recover. Resolution of these palsies is therefore directly related to the damage done at the time of injury.

The types of palsies are generally divided into injuries to the upper plexus (C5–C6 roots), Erb's palsy, or an injury to the lower plexus (C8 and T1 roots) Klumpke type, or a mixed pattern, in which all components of the plexus are involved, with generalized paralysis.

Clinically, in the upper type, or Erb's palsy, the Moro reflex is absent but grasp of the hand is present. In fact, the fingers and wrist have normal motion. The impaired muscles are the deltoid, the external rotators of the shoulder, elbow flexors and wrist extensors (supraspinatus, infraspinatus and teres minor, biceps brachii, brachialis, supinator, and the brachioradialis). The weakness results in a deformity in which the shoulder is adducted and internally rotated. The elbow is extended and the forearm pronated (the "waiter's tip position") (Figure 3.14). In the Klumpke type, or lower plexus injury, the limb also lacks a Moro reflex, and there is loss of grasp reflex. The wrist flexors, long digital flexors, and the intrinsic muscles of the hand are impaired, but the muscles controlling the shoulder and elbow are usually spared. The hand is supinated, the wrist extended, and the fingers clawed (Figure 3.15). In the mixed type of involvement, the limb is generally nearly flaccid. If a Horner's syndrome is seen in concert with a lower plexus injury, or a mixed type injury, the prognosis is guarded. From the primary care standpoint, the differential diagnosis includes fractures of the clavicle, injury to the proximal humeral epiphysis, infection of the upper humerus, and septic arthritis of the shoulder (Pearl 3.2). Radiographs of the cervical spine and shoulder are mandatory.

In spite of the severity of this problem, spontaneous recovery is common, with 85 percent of the cases regaining partial or full function by 18 months of age. The rapidity of recovery following birth seems directly related to the extent of the injury. It would seem logical for orthopedic referral to occur soon after recognition. Early treatment is concerned with maintaining a range of motion in those joints impaired by loss of motor control (stretching, positioning, splints). Once contractures or joint subluxation have occurred, surgical soft tissue releases, tendon transfers, and osteotomies become the front line of treatment protocols. Without question, the vast majority of cases seen are of the upper plexus, or Erb's palsy type, and remarkably few of these patients are substantially disabled enough to ever require surgical procedures. It has been observed that early return of elbow flexion (by six months of age) is directly related to more rapid and more extensive return of function in Erb's palsy. The overall incidence of brachial plexus injuries appears to be diminishing currently and is probably related to a much higher incidence of Cesarean section deliveries.

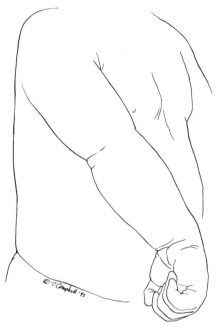

Figure 3.14. Characteristic position of the upper extremity in Erb's palsy.

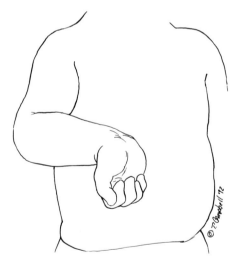

Figure 3.15. Characteristic upper extremity position in Klumpke's palsy.

Pearl 3.2. Differential diagnosis of birth palsies

Clavicle fractures
Proximal humerus fractures
Infection proximal humerus
Septic arthritis shoulder

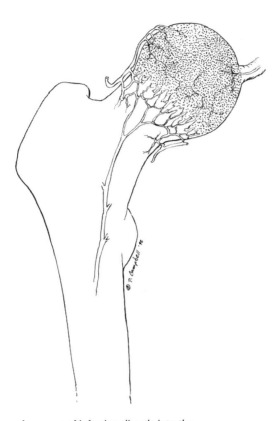

Figure 3.16. The ease of passage of infection directly into the chondroepiphysis due to the unique vascular arrangement in the infantile hip.

Figure 3.17. The rupturing of pus from a metaphyseal abscess into the joint with subsequent increased pressure and hip subluxation.

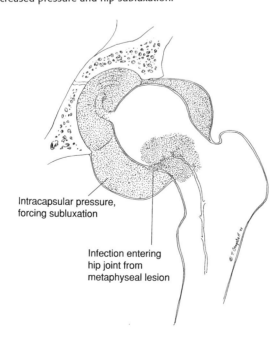

Intracapsular pressure, forcing subluxation

Infection entering hip joint from metaphyseal lesion

Septic arthritis of the hip

It is doubtful that the primary care physician will encounter an orthopedic condition, or injury, in children that bears such devastating sequelae as the consequences of inadequately managed septic arthritis of the hip. Even with seemingly appropriate management, there are times when disastrous consequences occur. Septic arthritis of the hip is best considered in two forms: an infantile form affecting the child from birth to the first year of life, and a later juvenile form. The infantile hip is separately characterized, primarily because it involves a hip in which the growth plate has not yet formed as an effective barrier between the metaphysis and the subsequent epiphysis. Infection residing within the metaphysis can easily extend directly across into the chondroepiphysis through vascular channels that have not yet been separated from the epiphysis (Figure 3.16). The infection within the metaphysis may also extend subperiostally, bursting directly into the hip joint itself, with the purulent fluid subsequently expanding within a contained space. As the infection progresses, the pressure within the hip joint capsule increases to a point where it may actually induce subluxation or dislocation of the hip (Figure 3.17). The infection spreading directly across into the chondroepiphysis may permanently impair the development of the secondary ossification center, and may permanently injure the developing growing cells of the future physis. In addition, the toxic by-products of the purulent exudate can act in a detrimental fashion on the cartilage of both the acetabulum and the chondroepiphysis. In the past it was not uncommon to see the femoral head completely resorbed as a consequence of a rampant untreated infection (Figure 3.18). Avascular necrosis of the femoral head, irreparable damage to the physis and the acetabular growth plate, arrest of the proximal femoral growth plate (Figure 3.19), chronic osteomyelitis, chronic subluxation, and dislocation of the hip are all highly undesirable sequelae.

In the juvenile form of septic arthritis of the hip, all of the previously noted sequelae may be present, with the exception that the growth plate acts as an effective barrier, usually preventing purulent material in the metaphysis from directly accessing the epiphysis. Instead, infection arising within the metaphysis will rupture beneath the periosteum and into the joint, thereby creating circulatory embarrassment and secondary pressure consequences to the femoral head. The origins of infection in the hip may arise from either direct hematogenous spread, or more commonly, from infection primarily originating within the metaphysis and then bursting into the hip joint itself.

In the face of such devastating complications, it is obvious that early recognition is the key to success. In the infantile form of septic arthritis, the child is usually irritable, fussy, and maintains the affected hip in a position of flexion, abduction, and external rotation (Figure 3.20). This position allows for the greatest amount of fluid to collect within the hip joint capsule without putting intense pressure on the very sensitive synovium. An increase in the intensity of the child's crying when the limb is moved into extension, abduction, or internal rotation should serve to demonstrate hip irritation. In the neonatal period, increased temperature and elevation of the sedimentation rate, elevated white blood count are often inconsistent, and may even delay diagnosis. Inasmuch as the ossification center of the femoral head does not generally appear until roughly three to six months of age, radiographs may only be helpful in showing some lateralization of the metaphysis of the femoral neck, or in demonstrating a lytic lesion within the metaphysis (Figure 3.21). The anteroposterior radiograph of the hip should be taken with the hips in a maximal position of extension with the knee in extension and the toes pointing directly upwards. Ultrasound can be extremely useful in documenting hip joint

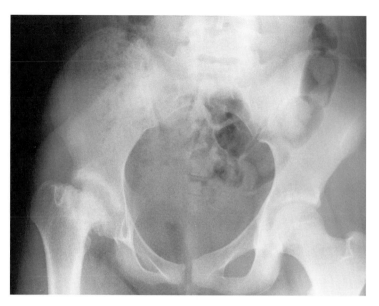

Figure 3.18. Anteroposterior radiograph demonstrating resorption of the femoral head as a consequence of septic arthritis.

Figure 3.19. Anteroposterior radiograph demonstrating avascular necrosis with growth plate closure, and arrest of femoral neck growth as sequelae of the septic arthritis of the hip.

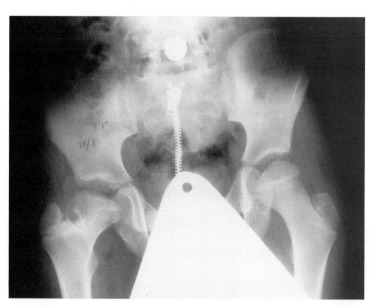

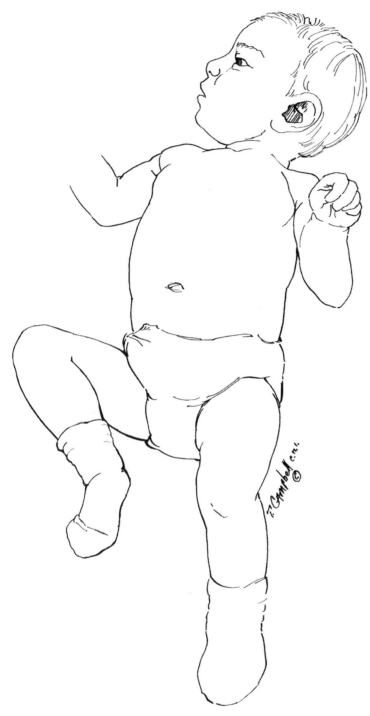

Figure 3.20. The characteristic position of the hip in acute septic arthritis.

effusion. Suspicion alone of a septic hip, in the infantile group, should be immediately followed by a needle aspiration of the hip joint.

Beyond the neonatal period, the clinical findings are identical; however, the sedimentation rate is routinely elevated (over 50 in near 90 percent of patients), and the temperature and white blood cell counts and C-reactive protein are usually elevated. Blood cultures are positive in roughly 50 percent of the cases. Any evidence of a lytic lesion in the metaphyseal neck, or widening of the joint space, in combination with the previously noted findings, should be followed by needle aspiration of the hip. Ultrasound commonly will demonstrate an effusion. If purulent material is recovered on needle aspiration of the hip, the optimal treatment is immediate surgical drainage of the infection. The condition should be treated as a surgical urgency/ emergency. Evacuation of all purulent material from the hip joint is necessary, and appropriate drainage should be carried out. Appropriate adjunct intravenous antibiotic therapy should be instituted in accordance with the recovery of an appropriate organism (Pearl 3.3) (Table 3.1).

In the infantile group of patients it has been estimated that over 50 percent will develop one or more of the consequences of an intraarticular infection in the future. These unsettling statistics should alert physicians to

Table 3.1 *Common organisms in childhood septic arthritis age/organism*

Age	Organism
Neonate	Streptococcus
	GM (-)
	Neisseria gonorrhea
Infant → 3 years	*Staphylococcus aureus*
	Haemophilus influenza
	Kingella kingae
>3 years	*Staphylococcus aureus*
Adolescents	*Staphylococcus aureus*
	Neisseria gonorrhea

consider this condition in every patient demonstrating hip irritation.

Congenital vertical talus

Perhaps the most rigid, and difficult to manage, congenital affectation of the musculoskeletal system in children is congenital vertical talus. A majority of the cases reported in the past, treated by competent practitioners, has resulted in disappointing outcomes. It is imperative that primary care physicians recognize and appreciate foot flexibility. Normally the foot and ankle can easily be mobilized through a full range of motion without evidence of joint stiffness. Stiffness is a characteristic of pathologic deformities of the foot, and is always present in congenital idiopathic clubfoot, and particularly in congenital vertical talus.

Congenital vertical talus is recognizable at birth and is most commonly confused with a calcaneal valgus postural foot deformity (Figure 3.22). The latter condition is a benign postural change that occurs as a consequence of the foot being compressed against the uterine wall. Spontaneous resolution is to be expected over the ensuing six months after birth. Congenital vertical talus is characterized by a *rigid* dorsiflexion deformity of the forefoot, and a fixed equinus of the hindfoot (Figure 3.23). The deformity has been termed a "rocker bottom foot or a Persian slipper" foot. This divergent deformity of hindfoot equinus and forefoot dorsiflexion produces considerable difficulties in management for the orthopedic surgeon.

In clinical practice roughly half of the cases seen are associated with other congenital and developmental syndromes, arthrogryposis, or most commonly, myelodysplasia. The condition should be readily recognizable if one constantly remembers the *rigidity* component. Once recognized, referral to a specialist orthopedic surgeon is advisable. Nearly all cases of congenital idiopathic vertical talus will

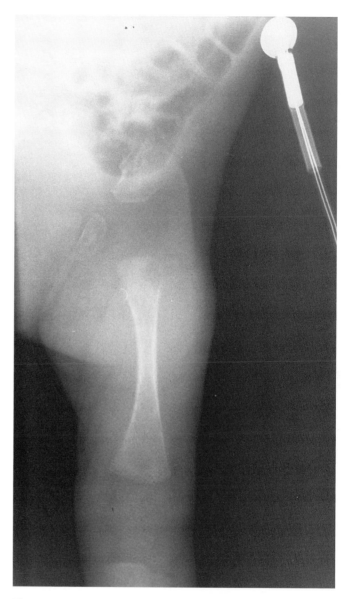

Figure 3.21. Anteroposterior radiograph demonstrating a lytic lesion in the femoral neck and subsequent septic subluxation of the hip.

Pearl 3.3. Diagnosis of septic arthritis hip

Clinical findings
↑Creactive protein
↑Sedimentation rate
↑White blood cells
+Blood culture
Needle aspiration
Radiographs

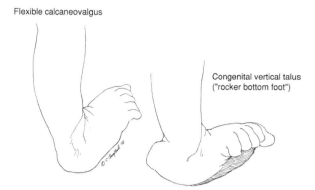

Figure 3.22. The differences in clinical picture between flexible calcaneus valgus foot and congenital vertical talus.

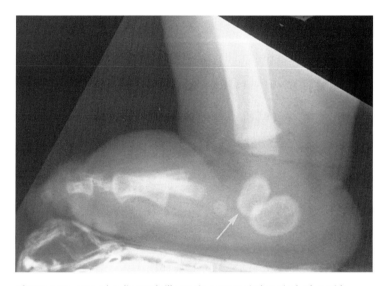

Figure 3.23. Lateral radiograph illustrating congenital vertical talus with equinus of the calcaneus and dorsiflexion of mid- and forefoot.

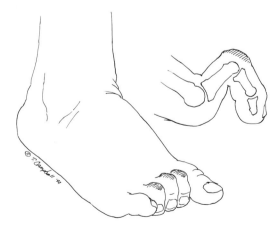

Figure 3.24. The clinical appearance of congenital hammer toe deformity.

require surgical procedures and orthopedic orthotic appliances. Encouraging aggressive surgical approaches have led to a greater success rate than previously experienced.

Congenital hammer toes

Congenital hammer toes are usually recognizable in the first year of life, and are routinely inherited. The "hammering" generally involves the second, third, and fourth toes. The distal interphalangeal joint is most commonly involved, but on occasion the proximal interphalangeal joint may be involved. The clinical appearance is characteristic and resembles a "hammer", by virtue of the distal phalanx being plantar flexed and rigid, relative to the middle phalanx, which lies in extension (Figure 3.24). Secondary to the rigidity, a painful corn commonly develops on the dorsal surface of the proximal or distal interphalangeal joint, precipitating medical attention. Symptomatic presentation usually occurs in the latter portion of the first decade to adolescence.

A protective sponge "donut" may be used over the painful corn to relieve discomfort temporarily, but most patients will eventually require more definitive procedures designed to straighten the affected joint and fuse it in a more desirable position. Surgical treatment should be reserved for those who have failed conservative care.

Congenital overlapping fifth toe

This condition is nearly always recognizable at birth, but may become more fully manifest symptomatically in the first two to three years of life. The fifth toe is dorsiflexed, adducted, and slightly externally rotated, and literally comes to lie on the dorsal surface of the fourth toe (Figure 3.25). Soft tissue contracture of the dorsal and medial structures of the fifth metatarsal phalangeal joint has been indicted as the cause of the deformity. Clinically, the toe not only lies dorsally and in an adducted position over the top of the fourth, but it cannot passively be reduced into its normal relationship. Those children who are symptomatic present with discomfort overlying the fifth toe with corns and painful calluses secondary to shoe wear. In general, surgical treatment should be reserved for only those cases in which substantial discomfort is present, and soft protective pads have failed. Most of the cases presenting with symptoms will eventually require surgical correction. Soft tissue releases, tendon rerouting, and metatarsophalangeal joint fusion provide the basis for reconstruction.

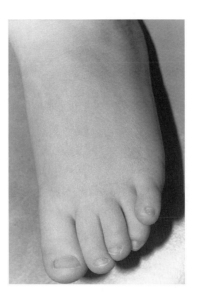

Figure 3.25. An overlapping fifth toe.

Supernumerary digits

Polydactyly, or supernumerary digits, is one of the most commonly seen congenital conditions in children. Most commonly the extra finger or toe is a mirror image of the digit lying directly adjacent to the extra digit (Figure 3.26). The apparent extra digit is in competition with the adjacent digit for the tendons activating that finger or toe. It is very important to determine tendon function in the presumed supernumerary digit so as not to become embarrassingly involved in the removal of a very functional part. The most common supernumerary digits are an extra fifth finger, an extra thumb, an extra fifth toe and an extra great toe. Not uncommonly, the extra thumb and toe will be syndactylized. Nearly always the indication for surgical removal is cosmetic, or as a consequence of difficulties in obtaining conventional shoe wear. Orthopedic referral is appropriate.

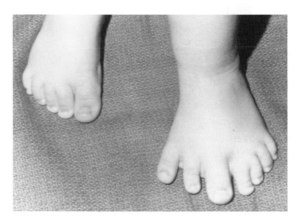

Figure 3.26. Supernumerary toes arising medial to the great toe.

Trigger thumb

Stenosing tenosynovitis of the thumb, more commonly known as "trigger thumb," is one of the more common congenital abnormalities of the hand. It is rarely recognized in the first six months of life since children generally maintain

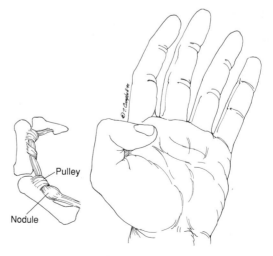

Figure 3.27. The clinical deformity and patho-anatomy of the trigger thumb.

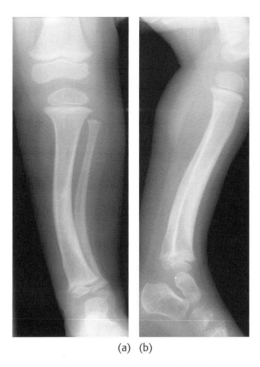

(a)   (b)

Figure 3.28. Anteroposterior (a) and lateral (b) radiographs of the tibia and fibula demonstrating medial (a) and posterior (b) bowing (posteromedial bowing).

Figure 3.29. (a) Anteroposterior radiograph showing lateral bowing of the tibia and fibula (anterolateral bowing). (b) Lateral radiograph demonstrating anterior bowing (anterolateral bowing).

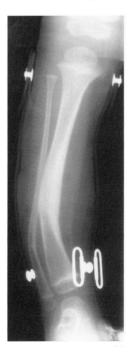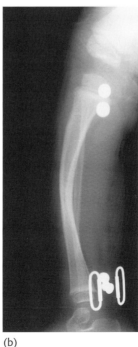

(a)   (b)

their hand in a fist-clenched position, and because they are not as yet using their hand for two-handed activities. As the child begins to reach, grasp, and grip objects, it becomes apparent that the thumb does not fully extend at the interphalangeal joint. The deformity may manifest itself in periodic episodes of flexion deformity of the interphalangeal joint with occasional episodes of popping, clicking or full straightening of the finger. More commonly it is recognized when the thumb is persistently held in a position of interphalangeal joint flexion (Figure 3.27). The parents relate that the thumb does not fully straighten, and that the child has some difficulty in grasping.

On examination, a palpable nodule is readily discerned at the metacarpophalangeal joint level, at or near the proximal metacarpophalangeal thumb crease. There is inability to extend the interphalangeal joint of the thumb. The palpable nodule is actually a thickened prominence arising from the flexor tendon to the thumb. As this nodule enlarges in size, it no longer is capable of passing through the flexor pulley, and complete extension of the thumb is impaired. Prior to the nodule reaching such size it may periodically pass through the tunnel, producing the characteristic "triggering" noticed by many parents.

Although stretching exercises and occasionally cortisone injections have been tried, the vast majority of children will require surgical release of the flexor pulley. Surgical treatment has routinely resulted in complete correction in well over 95 percent of the cases.

Congenital bowing of the tibia

Congenital bowing of the tibia is always recognizable at birth. It is most commonly seen unilaterally. Two forms are recognized: posteromedial bowing and anterolateral bowing. Congenital posteromedial bowing of the tibia produces a shortened leg from knee to ankle, with a posterior medial bow recognized at birth (Figures 3.28a, b). It is clearly the more benign of the two types of bowing of the tibia that are seen at birth. The natural evolution is benign as the posteromedial bowing gradually and spontaneously corrects over the ensuing years. The effectiveness of bracing in preventing fracturing is controversial (particularly since fractures almost never occur), although orthotic protection is commonly used. The limb is always shorter than the opposite side and the shortening, not uncommonly, leads to limb balancing surgical procedures during adolescence. Surgical considerations should not be entertained for the bowing itself.

Anterolateral bowing is a much more complex and much more treacherous deformity. Roughly half of the cases reported of anterolateral bowing of the tibia have occurred in association with either neurofibromatosis or fibrous dysplasia (Figures 3.29a, b). Anterolateral bowing of the tibia is generally considered under the terminology *congenital prepseudoarthrosis of the tibia*. Indeed many of the cases reported have already shown signs of an early fracture at the juncture of the upper two-thirds and lower third of the tibia. The bowing may be associated with a lytic type defect, fibrocystic in nature or neurofibrocystic in nature, at the site of the developing fracture or pseudoarthrosis, or the bowing may simply be associated with an obliteration of the medullary canal in the area of maximum bowing. In either case, the incidence of fracture is high, and the incidence of pseudoarthrosis is even greater. Cases in which the medullary canal is obliterated are usually managed by orthotics until maturity. Cases in which the fracture or fibrocystic pseudoarthrosis develops nearly always require surgical intervention. Complexities in obtaining acceptable surgical straightening and nonunion in this condition have resulted in innumerable below knee amputations, which must always be considered as a potential salvage in this condition (Pearl 3.4). Early recognition and appropriate orthopedic referral is indicated, particularly in light of

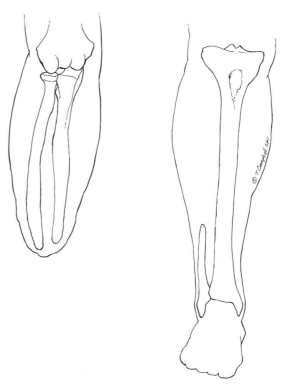

Figure 3.30. Drawing demonstrating terminal and intercalary limb absences.

Figure 3.31. Preaxial extremity long bones (radius and tibia) and postaxial extremity long bones (ulna and fibula).

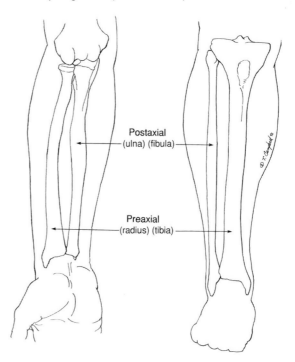

Postaxial
(ulna) (fibula)

Preaxial
(radius) (tibia)

Pearl 3.4. Prognosis in congential bowing of the tibia

"Good"
Posteromedial bow
"Bad"
Anterolateral bow
Neurofibromatosis
Pseudoarthrosis of tibia
Fibrous dysplasia

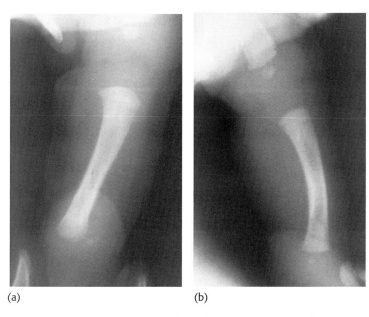

(a)   (b)

Figure 3.32. (a) Anteroposterior radiograph demonstrating complete absence of the fibula. (b) Lateral radiograph demonstrating complete absence of the fibula.

promising recent surgical advances (bone grafting techniques and skeletal fixation systems).

Juvenile amputee – congenital types

Juvenile amputees are generally classified as congenital or acquired. Further subdivision utilizes the term *terminal*, implying that the distal parts of the limb are absent and the remaining part has no terminal appendages. Intercalary implies that there is a proximal and a distal portion of the appendage present, but the interim portions are absent (Figure 3.30). The terms preaxial and postaxial refer to parts of the limb in which there are two bones, the radius and tibia being preaxial and the ulna and fibula postaxial (Figure 3.31). In general, congenital amputations resulting in partial or complete absence of a portion or all of a limb are managed by appropriate orthotics and prosthetics, commonly combined with surgical procedures to maximize functional potential.

Although congenital amputations are rare, the most common of these is *paraxial fibular hemimelia* or partial or complete absence of the fibula. In its most severe form, the entire fibula is absent as well as the lateral fourth and fifth rays of the foot (Figures 3.32a, b and 3.33). Commonly the talus and calcaneus are fused together. In all lower limb absences, there is always shortening of the limb, malrotation of the parts remaining, proximal joint instability, and proximal ligamentous and muscle aberrations. The only difference between the lower and upper extremity in this regard is the absence of prehensibility associated with the loss of hand function. In paraxial fibular hemimelia, there is commonly an eversion deformity of the foot and ankle (a reverse type of clubfoot deformity), and often instability at the level of the knee. In the more incomplete partial absences of the fibula, there may be little more than a short extremity and perhaps little need for any type of treatment; milder cases may show little more than simply a short leg from knee to foot. Treatment generally consists of limb length balancing, orthotic control, and occasionally surgical correction of the foot and ankle.

Proximal femoral focal deficiency is the second most common type of congenital lower limb absence. As with most congenital amputees, there is a wide variation in the type of cases seen, ranging from minimal alterations to severe deformity (Figure 3.34). The mildest form of proximal femoral focal deficiency results in a congenital short femur with some shortening of the limb, and perhaps some abnormalities in muscle and ligament stability and balance at the hip level. In the most severe form, the upper end of the femur as well as the acetabulum are absent. The children have a very short externally rotated flexed and abducted extremity, with a completely unstable pelvis and femur relationship. Nearly all cases of proximal femoral focal deficiency have severe limb shortening and will require efforts at limb balancing with orthotics or surgery and prosthetic management. The profound shortening and alteration in position of the femur make diagnosis obvious at birth.

Tibial hemimelia represents the least common form of the congenital lower limb absences. In its milder form, there is malrotation of the tibia, shortening of the limb, and usually an idiopathic clubfoot, associated with a reduction in tibial dimensions (Figure 3.35). In its most complete form, the tibia is absent; there is instability of the knee, severe shortening, and marked malrotation of the limb. Most cases of tibial hemimelia are associated with such a severe deformity of the leg from knee to foot that amputation is considered early. The severity of the deformity dictates the extent of treatment and the ultimate rehabilitation.

Although congenital absence of the digits of the upper extremity and even the hand itself may occur, the most commonly seen congenital absence of the upper extremity is congenital, partial, or complete absence of the

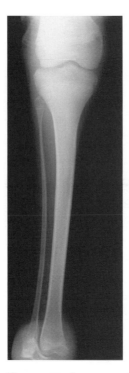

Figure 3.33. Anteroposterior radiograph demonstrating partial absence of the fibula.

Figure 3.34. Anteroposterior radiograph demonstrating severe and partial absence of the proximal femur.

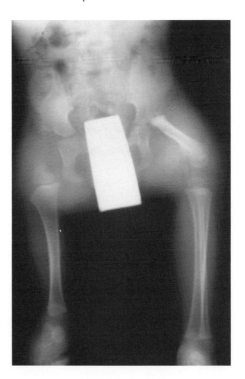

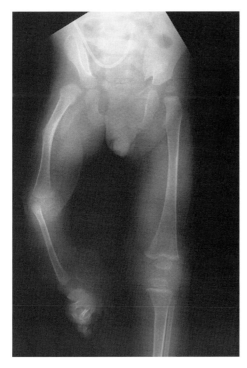

radius (Figure 3.36). It is not uncommonly bilateral, and in bilateral cases the association with Fanconi's anemia is well known. The thumb on the affected side is commonly hypoplastic or absent and the hand is deviated markedly toward the completely absent radius. The hand deformity is termed *radial clubhand*. It is readily recognizable at birth and early orthopedic referral is indicated. Early treatment commonly consists of appropriate orthotic splinting, followed by later reconstructive wrist stabilization.

Figure 3.35. Anteroposterior radiograph demonstrating complete absence of the tibia.

Figure 3.36. Radiograph demonstrating radial clubhand (partial absence of the radius).

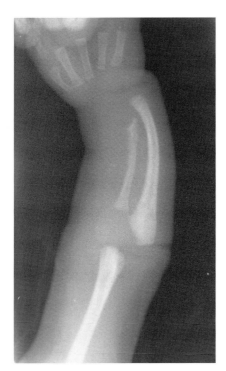

Chapter 4

From toddler to adolescence

A smarter mother often makes a better diagnosis than a poor doctor.

Bier

Idiopathic "toe-walking"

In the "early" walking period, "toe-walking" is one of the most common patterns troubling parents. The vast majority of patients presenting with "toe-walking" will spontaneously resolve with time and require only evaluation to eliminate other more serious causes. The idiopathic pattern of "toe-walking" will demonstrate a complete full range of ankle motion (dorsiflexion and plantar flexion) without any calf muscle contracture, but with walking an equinus position will be assumed. There may be some increased tone in the posterior calf muscles but as mentioned, the equinus posture disappears on examination.

More serious causes of "toe-walking" include cerebral palsy, muscular dystrophy, and congenital contracted (short) heelcords (Pearl 4.1). The differentiation by type is obviously important and will dictate the method of management. The primary care physician needs to be aware of the differential diagnoses and to seek orthopedic referral as necessary.

Pearl 4.1. Types of "toe-walking"

Idiopathic
Cerebral palsy
Muscular dystrophy
Congenital short heelcord

Juvenile myalgia ("growing pains")

Juvenile myalgia is probably the most appropriate term to represent a condition in children of remarkable prevalence. It is likely that parents of three siblings will have at least one child affected by this syndrome. In the past 50 years it has undergone a cyclic relegation from "old wives' tale" to a well-recognized condition. Although there is still profound disagreement concerning the etiology of this condition, it is highly likely that there is an organic basis for the reported symptoms, occurring characteristically at the end of the day in active youngsters. It is also highly likely that the by-products of muscle metabolism are implicated in the aching pain so commonly described by affected children. The syndrome is readily recognizable by the consistent nature of the symptoms, the total absence of clinically detectable abnormal orthopedic findings, and the absence of abnormal findings on laboratory investigation and radiographic assessment.

The condition is most commonly experienced between the ages of two and ten years with a peak age of roughly four to five years. Symptoms occur evenly in either sex and can occur unilaterally but more commonly are bilateral. They almost exclusively involve the lower extremities. The symptoms appear at the end of the day, in the early evening, or may even awaken the child at night. The condition presents as a dull, aching pain that characteristically is relieved by physical massage of the affected part, the application of heat, or the use of anti-inflammatory medications. With such modalities the symptoms will generally abate within a matter of minutes to hours, and will allow the child to return to a sleepful night. Children are generally not impaired during the daytime, and function as well as their peers. Parents deny the presence of swelling, redness, loss of motion, or any alteration that they can recognize in the affected part. It is common for the symptoms to last intermittently over a two-year period, punctuated by periods of exacerbation. The diagnosis is predicated on the classic history, and the total absence of clinical findings on either laboratory, radiography or physical

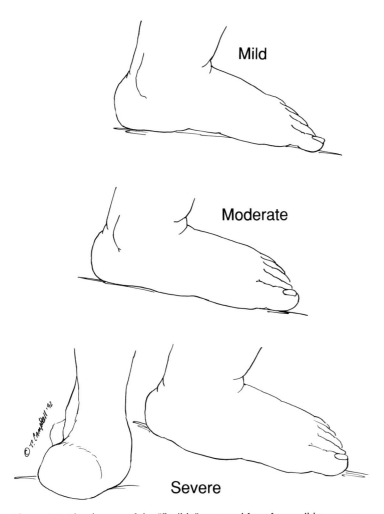

Figure 4.1. The degrees of the "flexible" pronated foot, from mild to severe.

examination. There is no limp, loss of motion, erythema, joint effusion, point tenderness, or abnormal limb attitudes. The symptoms have almost always been resolved by the latter part of the first decade. The treating physician should emphasize the benign prognosis of this condition and its ultimate resolution without sequelae.

The flexible pronated foot ("flexible flatfoot")

The term flexible pronated foot refers to a foot that on weight bearing assumes a position of apparent flattening of the medial longitudinal arch, or more properly, in-rolling of the ankle and eversion of the hindfoot. When weight bearing is removed (i.e., a child sitting over a table with the foot hanging free) an apparent longitudinal arch is present. Mild degrees of pronation of flattening of the longitudinal arch are recognized as a slight depression of the longitudinal arch with weight bearing with no substantial medial soft tissue bulging. Moderate pronation has generally been defined as flattening of the longitudinal arch to the floor with weight bearing with moderate protrusion of a soft tissue bulge (Figure 4.1). All of these observations are intrinsically subjective at best. Radiologic confirmation of degrees of pronation is nearly impossible in the age group in which the children present for management. The reason for this stems from the relatively immature degree of ossification of the bones of the foot in children between two and nine years of age. The difficulties in obtaining reproducible data on weight bearing radiographs will vary with: (1) the position of the foot on the X-ray plate relative to the incident beam of radiation; (2) inconsistency of reference points of measurement because of incomplete ossification of the foot; (3) varying the amount of pressure on the foot; and (4) variance in the degree of soft tissue present. The bones of the mid- and hindfoot ossify irregularly and present in differing shapes during various stages of growth. It is primarily for these reasons that this condition must be viewed as a clinical entity, rather than a radiographically documentable condition in the skeletally immature child.

In the past 50 years many millions of dollars have been spent on adaptive shoe wear and orthotic devices designed to change the structure of the developing longitudinal arch in children. In spite of this expenditure there is a profound absence of scientifically documented reports that have been able to establish that any alteration in the longitudinal arch in the skeletally immature youngster has occurred as a result of such devices. Furthermore, there is a substantial body of evidence that suggests that the flexible pronated adult is not disabled by the foot position. Even severe degrees of pronation no longer qualify one for military service exemption.

Our own experience in examining large numbers of pre-school and school age children, free of any foot complaints, has shown a correspondingly high incidence of longitudinal arch depression with weight bearing in the same age groups as those children presenting with parental complaints of "flatfoot." Physiologic valgus of the knees is most commonly encountered between the ages of three and seven years in children, and it is during these years that the highest prevalence of "flatfoot" presents to the primary care physician's office, or a pediatric orthopedist's office. A plethora of terms have been used to describe this condition, ranging from "hypermobile flatfoot," pronated foot, pes planus, pes planovalgus, pes valgus, flaccid flatfoot, and flexible plantar flexed talus. The term flexible pronated foot probably imparts the clearest visual perception of the clinical observations. It is interesting that to date there is not a single scientific study that has absolutely defined what constitutes a normal longitudinal arch. In most individuals axial loading of the mid- and hindfoot allows for a slight collapse into pronation with the hindfoot tilting into valgus. In the most severe forms of flexible pronated feet there is commonly a family history, and not uncommonly, an associated generalized ligamentous laxity. Studies have shown that the human longitudinal arch may not be fully formed until six or seven years of age at the earliest. In children under 12 years of age, a painful foot associated with pronation should influence the examiner to exclude such conditions as tarsal coalition, contracted heelcord, tarsal osteochondritis, posterior tibial tendonitis with accessory navicular, juvenile arthritis, and calcaneal apophysitis.

All imaginable forms of treatment for the flexible pronated foot have at one time or another been utilized, including surgical methods. With the exception of surgery there is a generalized lack of scientific documentation that devices alter the natural evolution of these flexible pronated feet. Furthermore, it is almost impossible to imagine that a static device worn during the "walking" portion of one's day would substantially influence the formation
of the composite soft tissues and bony arch, which are likely under genetic controls as well.

Children with flexible pronated feet are most commonly brought to the physician's office because of concern over the cosmetic appearance of the foot, excessive use of shoe wear, and only occasionally in the adolescent, with foot pain. It must be remembered that by skeletal age 13 years, nearly 90 percent of the foot has matured (females earlier than males). Parents commonly have been conditioned to expect some sort of treatment for their concerns, and it is far easier to prescribe an adaptive shoe or a prescription orthosis than it is to take the time and energy to explain to parents and convince them that treatment is unnecessary. Diagnosis rests with the observable predescribed findings combined with the exclusion of any pathologic foot condition. Radiographs are generally unnecessary unless another condition is suspected, or there is undue parental concern. Treatment in any form is universally successful and nearly universally unnecessary. In light of available current knowledge, the flexible pronated foot most likely represents a variant of "normal."

Transient (toxic) synovitis of the hip in children

Transient synovitis of the hip is one of the most common hip disorders in childhood, far more common than Legg–Calvé– Perthes disease, and characterized by the acute onset of a painful limp or inability to bear weight. The typical presentation is that of a child between 4 and 10 years of age, who awakens in the morning with pain in the area of the thigh region or the knee, and who resists weight bearing. Attempts to rotate the hip internally, abduct the hip, and fully extend the hip are generally met with discomfort. The ratio of males to females is roughly two to one in favor of males, and in well over two-thirds of the cases a history of a premonitory upper respiratory tract infection can be obtained. Laboratory work and radiographs are usually within normal limits.

The temperature may be mildly elevated, and the white blood count and sedimentation rate also may be mildly elevated. C-reactive protein levels are generally normal. Radiographs generally reveal no bony alterations, although occasionally some widening of the hip joint space or mild osteopenia may be detected. Radionuclide imaging will usually show a synovitis type pattern. Ultrasound evidence of intraarticular fluid fails to distinguish transient synovitis of the hip from septic arthritis. In cases where septic arthritis is suspected, needle aspiration of the affected hip will be particularly helpful in differentiation. Aspirations of hips affected with transient synovitis have rarely shown any abnormal laboratory changes and cultures will be negative. The actual diagnosis is largely a diagnosis of exclusion (Pearl 4.2). The etiology of transient synovitis is still unclear. The clinical

---

Pearl 4.2. Differential diagnosis

Transient synovitis hip
Clinical findings
Mild ↑ sedimentation rate
Mild ↑ WBC (white blood cells)
Normal CRP (C-reactive protein)
⊖ Aspirate
⊖ Blood culture
Septic arthritis hip
Clinical findings
Sedimentation rate > 50
↑ WBC
↑ CRP
⊕ Aspirate
⊕ Blood culture

course most closely parallels that of an allergic response to perhaps a bacterial or viral antigen.

In general, the overall prognosis is quite good, with symptoms resolving in a matter of days to a few weeks. Conservative treatment consisting of periodic bed rest, and occasional traction, has routinely resulted in resolution of symptoms. Recurrences of symptoms are not uncommon and may occur in up to 10 to 15 percent of cases. The major differential diagnosis of recurrent cases rests between Legg–Calvé–Perthes disease and juvenile rheumatoid arthritis. Because a few cases have eventually shown evidence of avascular necrosis, and a few have exhibited more clear findings of juvenile rheumatoid arthritis, it is suggested that the children be followed for a few months after the disease appears to have clinically resolved. In spite of these occasional and more serious later developments, the overall prognosis is benign in most cases.

Benign migratory rheumatism is an older term that has been used to describe what most likely is a form of transient synovitis of the knee. It is not uncommon in practice to find children between the ages of two and six years in whom the parents have identified a limp on arising in the morning, and then gradually resolving with activities of the day. The parents characteristically will refer to discomfort in the knee or the ankle and may even relate a story of swelling about the knee. Although an antalgic/painful type limp is commonly seen on physical examination, there is only rarely an effusion of the knee, and even rarer is there restriction of motion of the knee. Most commonly a descriptive story of the painful early morning limp is all that is available for diagnosis, as clinical findings are unusual. Although the condition bears some resemblance to juvenile rheumatoid arthritis by history, it has a very favorable benign prognosis. Symptoms generally resolve within a one to two year period and recurrences are exceedingly uncommon. Treatment is at best supportive, with reassurance to the parents all that is necessary.

Legg–Calvé–Perthes disease

The patient with Legg–Calvé–Perthes disease presents with a limp, usually of the antalgic or painful type, and commonly made worse with activities. The limp generally reflects hip irritation or synovitis and very importantly is not directly related to the degree of radiographic changes evident in the femoral head. If Legg–Calvé–Perthes disease is verified on the radiographs the leg is usually shorter, and there may be some thigh atrophy as a reflection of disuse, secondary to discomfort. Not uncommonly the hip will be restricted in its range of motion, particularly in hip abduction and internal rotation. All children exhibiting signs of hip irritation demand radiographic evaluation. Plain radiographs are capable of establishing a diagnosis in well over 95 percent of all cases. Only occasionally has radionuclide imaging been found necessary when clear-cut radiographic changes were not evident. The most commonly seen changes in association with Legg–Calvé–Perthes disease are a widening of the medial joint space, a subchondral crescent sign (or subchondral fracture) seen in the weight bearing anterosuperior and lateral aspect of the femoral head, irregular changes in the density of the head, fragmentation of the ossified portion of the head, a vertical reduction in height of the epiphysis, and not uncommonly, a lateral extrusion of the femoral head from the confines of the acetabulum (Figures 4.2a, b; 4.3; 4.4). The diagnosis is therefore suspected clinically and established radiographically. Orthopedic surgical referral is recommended at that point in time.

Our preoccupation with the uncommon and fascinating is strikingly crystallized in the literature on Legg–Calvé–Perthes disease. Over 20 times the number of English-speaking articles on this condition have been published for every article on transient synovitis of the hip. This is a clear paradox of interest, since the physician will likely encounter cases of

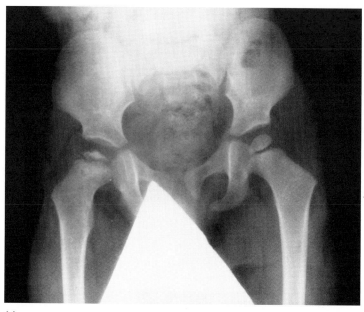

(a)

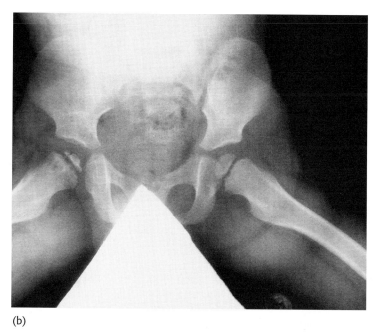

(b)

Figure 4.2. Anteroposterior (a) and lateral (b) radiographs demonstrating early Legg–Calvé–Perthes disease with total head involvement.

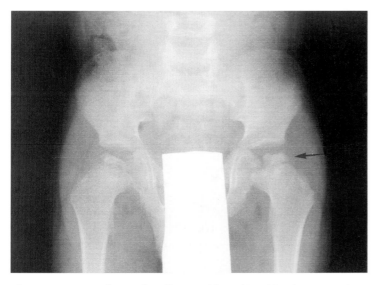

Figure 4.3. Legg–Calvé–Perthes disease with total head involvement and more advanced changes of femoral head fragmentation.

Figure 4.4. Anteroposterior radiograph demonstrating advanced stage of femoral head deformity secondary to Legg–Calvé–Perthes disease.

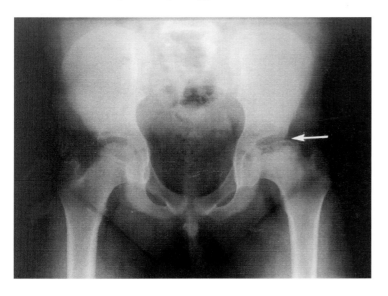

transient synovitis of the hip at least four to five times more commonly.

Although we have learned a great deal about the natural history of treated and untreated Legg–Calvé–Perthes disease, we have added little of significance to our understanding of the basic etiology since 1907 when Legg in Boston, Calvé in France, and Perthes in Germany gained the honor of the original descriptions. Legg, in fact, suggested that he was unsure that treatment would ever affect the natural history of this disease, and now over 90 years later, we have improved our overall results with treatment only moderately (20 to 30 percent improved radiographic results).

Although the exact etiology still evades our understanding, the overwhelming body of evidence would suggest that this condition is a generalized constitutional disorder of growth. A certain type of child is most susceptible (i.e., male, blue-eyed, light fine hair, alert, active, shorter in stature than expected norms, and between 4 and 10 years of age). It is likely that the radiographic hip changes merely reflect the capital femoral epiphysis' susceptibility and fragility to unknown insults to its blood supply. Nearly 90 percent of the cases show retardation of the bone age of a significant nature. The final common pathway of the unknown etiologic factors is avascular necrosis of the femoral capital epiphysis, in part or full. Biopsies have substantiated that while cellular death of the epiphysis is always present; there is always demonstrable healing, with reparative bone occurring simultaneously, to a greater or lesser degree. This biologic ingrowth of revascularized tissue prevents the actual loss of bone substance seen so commonly in elderly people with avascular necrosis. The femoral head always recovers, and although it may substantially deform, it does not disappear.

The evolutionary end result of this "death and healing" process is a femoral head that is relatively spherical (normal) or deformed in degrees, with the worst result being a flattened expanded head with a short squat femoral neck, and a high-riding greater trochanter. Three basic radiographic patterns have been described to characterize the end result hip: spherical congruity (a round ball with a round socket); aspherical congruity (a deformed ball with an accommodating deformed socket); and aspherical incongruity (a squared flat type ball with a round socket) (Figure 4.5). It has been shown that aspherical incongruity will most regularly result in the greatest number of cases with premature arthritis requiring total hip replacement or other reconstructive surgery in the future.

Once the femoral head begins to extrude outside the confines of the outer ledge of the acetabulum, and if the healing process within the head is incomplete, the head will continue to deform (flatten) and permanently become misshapen, leading to a much greater risk of eventual arthritis. Treatment is designed to intercede and arrest this "extrusion" process, as mild degrees of deformity are often seen to reshape and remodel, and often retain a spherical contour. From the patient's standpoint the basic issue is rather simple: is premature arthritis likely to occur, and can any form of treatment prevent it? Currently most orthopedic surgeons have embraced the concept of "containment." Containment embraces the concept that during loading of the femoral head (i.e., walking, running, jumping), the head be kept totally within the confines of the acetabulum so that the "biologically plastic" or deformable femoral head can be molded into a spherical shape, and that a portion of the head will not "bulge" or extrude from the margins of the acetabulum.

Consequently most currently popular forms of treatment seek to achieve, by one technique or another, containment of the head within the socket. Reducing weight-bearing (i.e., using crutches) has not been shown to improve overall results nor does it provide containment. Surgically this is accomplished by directing the upper part of the femur more deeply into the acetabulum (femoral osteotomy), or rotating the acetabulum itself to further cover the head

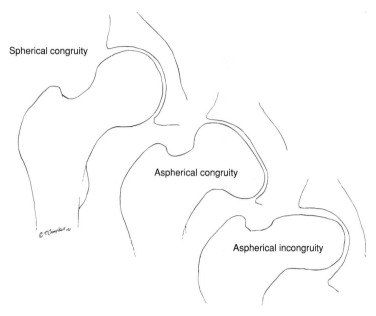

Spherical congruity

Aspherical congruity

Aspherical incongruity

Figure 4.5. The various degrees of hip joint congruency/ incongruency.

(a)

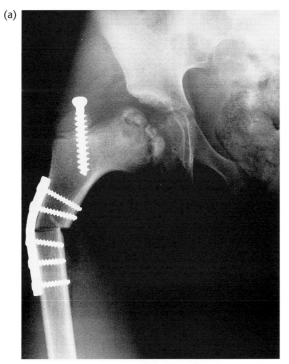

(b)

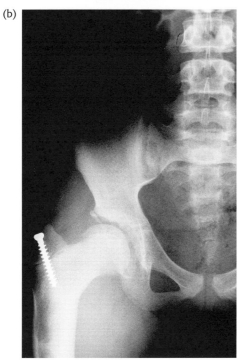

Figure 4.6. (a) Anteroposterior radiograph demonstrating femoral head containment following varus osteotomy of the proximal femur.
(b) Anteroposterior radiograph showing femoral neck-shaft remodeling and femoral head remodeling, following osteotomy of the proximal femur for Legg–Calvé–Perthes disease.

(innominate osteotomy). Those who believe in bracing seek the same end point, but rely on the brace and the patient's *compliance* to wear the brace, a difficult process at best, to maintain the head in the contained position. Proponents of surgical techniques argue that the treatment time is reduced to roughly three to four months as compared to an average of two to three years with the bracing technique (Figures 4.6a, b). Conversely, proponents of bracing argue that the bracing avoids an operation, and that results are comparable. From recent radiographic evidence, surgery has a far greater percentage of satisfactory outcomes compared to other treatment techniques. The role of primary care physicians is to be aware of the various treatment selections available to their patients and to provide appropriate referral in all stages of active disease.

Osteomyelitis

Osteomyelitis is an infection in bone, most frequently occurring in infants and young children, although it may be observed at any age during childhood. It is more common in males by a three to one ratio for reasons unknown. The current incidence is 1 in 5000. A slightly higher incidence is noted in late summer and early fall. Most commonly, the source of bone infection is from hematogenous spread, but there are also cases of direct extension from soft tissue, and by the external introduction of infection. A history of recent trauma is often elicited prior to onset. As a classic example, the metaphysis of the long bones, because of its peculiar anatomy and profuse blood supply, is the most common site of inoculation. The infecting organisms reach the metaphysis through the nutrient vessel supply. The nutrient artery in the metaphysis eventually empties into a large sinusoidal system with a reduced rate of blood flow. This sluggish circulation is believed to provide an enhanced atmosphere for the proliferation of pathogenic bacteria, and for the abscess to be nurtured and enlarged in dimension. A paucity of immune cells in the area may also contribute to progression. As the abscess enlarges it creates areas of increased localized pressure secondary to the fluid pressure within, and subsequently affects the nutrition to the adjacent bony trabeculae. The increasing head of pressure within the abscess allows the infection to extend within the metaphysis and out through the Volkmann's canals to gain access to the subperiosteal space, where the periosteum may actually become elevated (Figure 4.7). If left uncontrolled, the infection may rupture through the periosteum permitting pus to escape into the soft tissues. The abscess can readily extend up and down the shaft into the diaphysis. In children under 18 months of age, where the physis has not yet been formed as a barrier between the metaphysis and the epiphysis, the infection can readily extend across the future growth plate and affect both the growth plate and the growing epiphysis. In bones in which the metaphysis lies within a joint, subperiosteal rupture can lead to direct extension into the joint and produce septic arthritis (Figure 4.8). The hip, shoulder, ankle and elbow (radial head) serve as examples of such extrusion. Patients with reduced immunity, sickle cell disease, and organ transplant patients are known to be particularly susceptible.

Although systemic symptoms of fever, chills, reduced appetite, and malaise are often present, pain is the most striking clinical feature. In addition to systemic symptoms, the pain is generally localized, and is believed to be the result of the expanding abscess causing pressure on local nerves. Fine nerve fibrils are present in association with vascular channels in the metaphyses. The child is reluctant to move the affected limb or joint, and an antalgic limp is common. In the newborn and very young, the child may be merely irritable, refuse feeding, and show reduced limb movement (pseudoparalysis). Palpation over the affected metaphyseal region will nearly always result in acute exacerbation of the painful symptoms. If

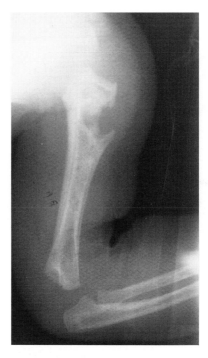

Figure 4.7. Radiograph demonstrating an abscess with marked periosteal reaction secondary to suppurative osteomyelitis.

Figure 4.8. Penetration of an abscess into hip joint from metaphysis with ensuing subluxation.

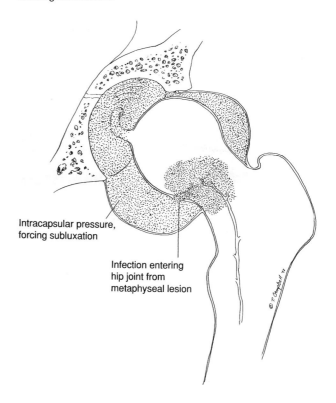

Intracapsular pressure, forcing subluxation

Infection entering hip joint from metaphyseal lesion

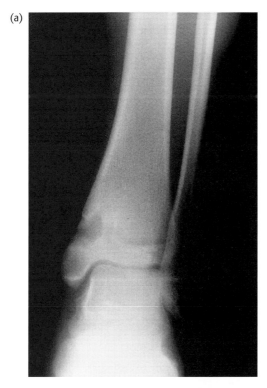

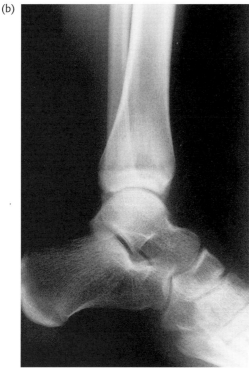

Figure 4.9. Anteroposterior (a) and lateral (b) radiographs demonstrating osteomyelitic abscess of the distal tibia.

a particular area is suspected, the clinical examination should preserve that area toward the end of the examination to avoid exacerbating the patient's response prematurely. Localized erythema and edema are common.

Radiographically, changes within the bone substance are rarely seen before 7–10 days after the initial infection and abscess is forming. During these initial 7–10 days, areas of soft tissue swelling and regional areas of osteopenia are all that may be seen on radiographs. After 7–10 days following the initial infection, areas of rarefaction or established lysis may appear on the radiograph, representing resorbed trabeculae secondary to the localized abscess (Figures 4.9a, b). At the same time, or shortly afterwards, periosteal new bone formation may appear, reflecting the transit of infection into the subperiosteal region. Advanced cases may show an area of sequestered dead bone appearing as dense bone and may even show an involucrum, or the new layer of reparative bone surrounding the sequestrum. As early as 24–48 hours following the initial abscess formation, radionuclide bone scanning may be useful in localizing the abscess. Although the findings are nonspecific, the accuracy rates in predicting osteomyelitis have been estimated to be up to 90 percent. Magnetic resonance imaging (MRI) may be useful in identifying an abscess when antibiotics have been ineffective or when other imaging has failed to provide a diagnosis. Well-known alterations in peripheral white blood count culture, sedimentation rate, C-reactive protein, and identification of the offending organism are obvious important diagnostic adjuncts. C-reactive protein may be particularly useful, as it is typically the first parameter to increase in response to infection and in following the response to antibiotics.

Commonly the site of the affected bony metaphysis becomes locally tender and hyperemic. It is therefore important to consider introducing a needle into the metaphysis, both for diagnostic purposes and to retrieve the offending organism if possible. In fact if osteomyelitis is a strong consideration, needle aspiration should be considered in nearly every circumstance. Delaying antibiotic therapy is desirable to identify organisms through blood cultures and needle aspiration.

It is extremely important that both primary care physicians and orthopedic surgeons work in synchrony in the assessment and management of a child with osteomyelitis. Prior to radiographic evidence of localized rarefaction within the bone substance, appropriate antibiotics may be all that is necessary. Once radiographic evidence of rarefaction or lysis within the bone is apparent, surgical evacuation of the infectious process is generally indicated. During the neonatal period, Group B streptococcus and gram-negative enteric bacilli seem to be the most prevalent organisms, although *Staphylococcus aureus* may also be seen. Beyond the neonatal period and into the toddler years, *S. aureus* and *Hemophilus influenzae* become more prevalent (see Table 3.1). However, clinical infection with the *H. influenzae* has dramatically receded with the widespread use of the vaccine. In the management of osteomyelitis, failure of systemic antibiotics to result in a relatively rapid change in temperature, localized tenderness, and overall well-being within a 48-hour period should lead one to consider surgical decompression, particularly in the case of a positive bone aspiration. Certainly the presence of purulent material on aspirate combined with radiographic evidence of rarefaction should lead to operative intervention. Surgical decompression is designed to immediately evacuate the abscess and provide a drainage conduit for any re-accumulating purulent material.

Other than the well-known complication of chronic osteomyelitis developing from an inadequately treated primary infection, children are also susceptible to other late sequelae. These include local insult to the growth plate, resulting in angular or rotational deformity, shortening, or overgrowth of the extremity. Occasionally a "burned-out" latent abscess cavity (Brodie's abscess) may develop subsequently and reactivate at a later time. In very young children, the metaphyseal abscess may extend directly across the physis and involve the epiphysis. The weakened metaphyses may be subject to pathologic fracture, and even displacement of the entire epiphysis and growth plate has been reported. Urgent diagnosis and appropriate treatment will obviate the need for management of potentially devastating late sequelae.

Septic arthritis

Although septic arthritis in the very young child has been previously described, it is important to remember that it can occur in all age groups from toddler to adolescence. *Hemophilus influenzae* is a common organism in the toddler age group, but from age three years onward *S. aureus* becomes the most prevalent organism. Initially the infecting organism produces a synovial reaction of edema, hyperemia, and an increased amount of synovial fluid. As the infection progresses, frank purulent material accumulates within the joint cavity, and by a combination of the intraarticular increase in pressure, combined with local destructive changes induced by the infecting organism (lysozyme mediated), actual destruction of the articular cartilage may occur. The increased pressure within the joint not only can cause local destructive changes in the soft tissues and cartilage surfaces, but may also result in joint subluxation or dislocation.

The clinical picture is usually rather obvious, with severe pain at all attempts to manipulate the joint, joint stiffness, erythema, and edema. In the lower extremity the child will have a pronounced limp or will fail to bear weight at all. Systemic manifestations of infection are generally present.

Although laboratory studies and radionuclide imaging may be helpful and ultrasound may be useful in documenting intraarticular effusion, direct needle aspiration of the joint is the single most important diagnostic tool (Pearl 4.3). Joint aspiration, in the absence of prior antibiotics, will often provide evidence of a bacterial infection, and culture of the affecting organism will lead the clinician to appropriate antibiotic therapy. The most common differential dilemma is in discerning juvenile rheumatoid arthritis from nonbacterial synovitis.

In most cases surgical drainage of the septic arthritis is indicated to evacuate the purulent material. Surgical drainage is performed always in conjunction with appropriate antibiotic therapy. The peculiar anatomy of the hip in the child under 18 months of age renders the hip particularly susceptible to the consequences of joint infection. Intraarticular abscess may occlude the blood supply to the physis, damage the articular cartilage of the femoral head and acetabulum and impair the future growth and development of the head and acetabulae, and induce stretching of the capsule and chronic subluxation or dislocation of the hip. In very advanced cases, the hip joint may be destroyed by resorption of the upper femur (Figure 4.10). Septic arthritis of the hip demands urgent or emergent decompression, and appropriate therapy. The sequelae of hip joint infection are disastrous, but septic arthritis of other joints may be equally disabling, resulting in joint destruction with stiffness and chronic pain. A rapid, aggressive, early diagnosis and treatment plan is imperative.

Disc space infection

Disc space infection (discitis), is by far most commonly seen in children between the toddler and adolescent years, and is found equally in males and females. Disc space infection commonly affects children younger than five years of age but can occur in any age group. In spite of the rather dramatic symptoms and findings, the prognosis overall is generally

Pearl 4.3. Diagnosis of septic arthritis hip

Clinical findings
↑C-reactive protein
↑Sedimentation rate
↑White blood cells
+ Blood culture
Needle aspiration
Radiographs

Figure 4.10. Anteroposterior radiograph demonstrating severe destructive changes in the femoral head and neck secondary to septic arthritis.

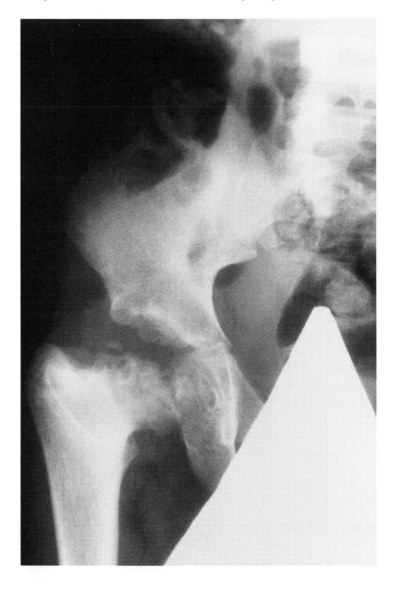

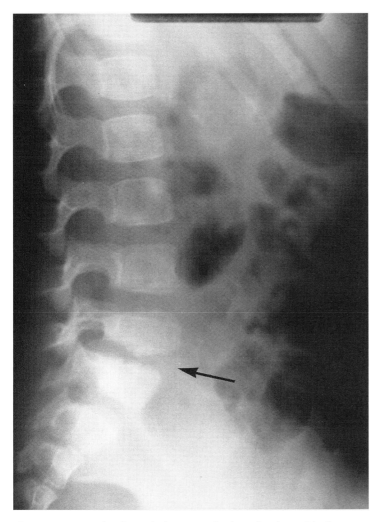

Figure 4.11. Lateral radiograph demonstrating irregular changes in the vertebral end plates, sclerosis, and narrowing of the intervertebral disc seen in disc space infection.

Pearl 4.4. Sailent features of "discitis"

Severe back pain
"Splinting"
Radiographs
⊕ Bone scan
Marked ↑ Sedimentation rate

---

quite good. The cornerstone of symptoms is the intense back pain encountered by patients. Occasionally the localization of the back pain may be somewhat vague, particularly in young children, with aching pain radiating into the buttocks and posterolateral thighs. Localized lumbar symptoms are most common, and children will refuse to walk, refuse to sit, and refuse to be manipulated. Young children may or may not be febrile, and rarely will show severe malaise or lack of appetite.

On examination any movements that elicit motion adjacent to the affected vertebral disc space will cause immediate "splinting" and discomfort. A useful clinical test is to invite the child to "pick up" a toy on the floor and then observe "splinting." Radiographs characteristically reveal a reduction in the vertical height of the disc space, irregularity of the vertebral end plates, and changes in density (Figure 4.11). Computed tomography scanning and magnetic resonance imaging may be helpful as well, but are usually unnecessary. Radionuclide imaging most commonly will show an intense uptake adjacent to the vertebral end plates of the affected disc space. The sedimentation rate is nearly always significantly elevated, and is often the only laboratory test abnormality. Many patients are afebrile. Magnetic resonance imaging may be useful in complicated diagnosis or occasionally when epidural abscess is suspected. Disc space aspiration has been successful in retrieving the affecting organism only 50 percent of the time, and is not routinely performed. Radionuclide imaging is extremely useful in establishing diagnosis (Pearl 4.4).

One of the most interesting features of the disease rests with the fact that if supportive treatment alone is used (pain medication, back splinting by bed rest, plaster, or plastic splints, relief from weight bearing), the results are nearly always successful. Although antibiotic therapy is commonly used, generally to combat *S. aureus*, it is not generally believed to be essential for treatment but may occasionally shorten the clinical course. For reasons as yet unclear, the affected disc space and its surrounding vertebrae seem capable of containing and eradicating the infectious organism in virtually all cases. Cases of retrograde extension of an abscess or anterior extradiscal extravasation are very rare. Inasmuch as symptoms commonly continue for four to six weeks after the initial episode, continual supportive care and observation are important. Patients who are immunosuppressed are most susceptible to this condition. Tuberculosis can be occasionally encountered. The high index of suspicion in the primary care physician, coupled with the dramatic nature of the presenting symptoms and findings, should lead one readily to the diagnosis. Orthopaedic referral is appropriate.

Juvenile rheumatoid arthritis

Rheumatoid arthritis in children is a systemic disorder that generally presents in one of three different patterns. The systemic multisystem disease with generalized arthritis (Still's disease) is probably the least common form seen in children. Pauciarticular arthritis and polyarthritis without marked systemic changes are far more common. The greatest concentration of cases will occur during the toddler to adolescent years, with the prevalence greatest between five and eight years of age.

Although the exact etiology of juvenile rheumatoid arthritis is unclear, it is generally perceived to be an autoimmune disorder, in which an inflammatory factor within the joint causes the release of lysosomal enzymes, with resultant damage to the articular surfaces of the joint. Whatever the nature of the etiology, the synovial joints reflect the inflammatory process more than any other structure. As the synovium becomes inflamed it produces excessive joint fluid, but the fluid produced is thin and "watery" with an inadequate amount of mucin. The synovium proliferates and may form nodules and thickened villi that project into the

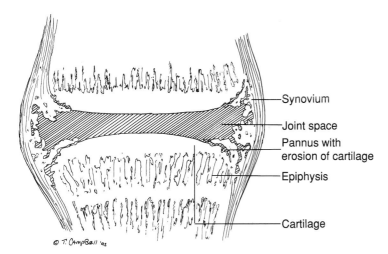

Synovium

Joint space

Pannus with erosion of cartilage

Epiphysis

Cartilage

© T. Campbell '92

Figure 4.12. The proliferative synovitis seen in juvenile rheumatoid arthritis with the "pannus" producing articular cartilage erosion.

joint space. Further proliferation may result in the pannus forming over the articular cartilage, depriving the cartilage of its normal diffusion of nutrients, and an increased amount of fibrosis both within the joint and in the pericapsular and capsular structures (Figure 4.12).

Eventually the nutrition to the articular cartilage is sufficiently impaired that cartilage degradation ensues, with resulting arthritis. Restriction in the joint capsule and ligaments results in increasing limitations of joint motion. Adjacent and distant tendons may become involved with the reactive synovial inflammation, leading to chronic tendonitis, tendon destruction, and even tendon rupture. Although uncommon, "rheumatoid" nodules, particularly on the extensor surfaces of the elbows and knee, may appear. Synovial biopsies have not been found to be specifically diagnostic of juvenile rheumatoid arthritis.

The most severe form of rheumatoid arthritis in children (Still's disease) is most commonly seen at onset prior to the toddler age group. The cervical spine may be involved and joint instability may ensue. The most common type seen during the toddler to adolescent range is the pauciarticular type of arthritis. Most commonly the joints of the lower extremities are affected, with the knee being the most frequent site. In roughly one half of the cases involvement is monoarticular, and in roughly 25 percent of the cases two joints are affected. Females seem to be affected nearly twice as commonly as males. Clinically children in this age group are systemically ill, but more commonly present with a limp, and an erythematous or "swollen" joint with restricted motion and pain. Characteristically the symptoms are far worse in the morning, and as the children become more active during the day the symptoms recede. Local findings of erythema, warmth, restriction of motion, and joint effusion are seen.

Commonly the erythrocyte sedimentation rate is elevated and radionuclide imaging may show a synovitis type pattern. Joint aspiration is of value particularly in differentiating this

Table 4.1 *Synovial fluid analysis inflammatory/infectious*

Appearance	Inflammatory Clear yellow/green	Infectious Cloudy/creamy
WBC	<60,000	>50,000
Viscosity	Dec.	Dec.
Mucin	Poor	Poor
Bacteria	⊖	⊕
Glucose	Normal	↓

condition from suppurative arthritis (Table 4.1). Ophthalmologic evaluations should be obtained in all cases of pauciarticular juvenile rheumatoid arthritis because of the incidence of uveitis, which may be present in 15–20 percent of cases.

In the absence of uveitis, the prognosis of pauciarticular juvenile rheumatoid arthritis is overall quite good, with over two-thirds of the cases resolving or with minimal joint disabilities. Patients with polyarticular involvement with minimal systemic manifestations and multiple joint involvement appear to have a peak incidence between eight and ten years of age, particularly in females. The findings are similar to all other types, with warm, tender, painful joints and a history of morning stiffness (Figure 4.13). Involvement of the ankles and feet, joints of the fingers, cervical spine, and temporomandibular joints are commonly seen. The prognosis in this form of juvenile arthritis is somewhat worse than pauciarticular, but not as severe as the classic systemic disease with polyarthritis (Still's disease).

Radiographic evaluation in rheumatoid arthritis in children may demonstrate soft tissue swelling, capsular distention, and relative osteopenia in the periarticular regions. All of the changes seen are nonspecific in nature. Only in the very advanced stages of articular cartilage destruction does evidence of joint narrowing and subchondral erosions appear (Figure 4.14). Epiphyseal and physeal growth may be accelerated or retarded. Appropriate anti-inflammatory medications in

Figure 4.13. Swollen knee joint seen in juvenile rheumatoid arthritis.

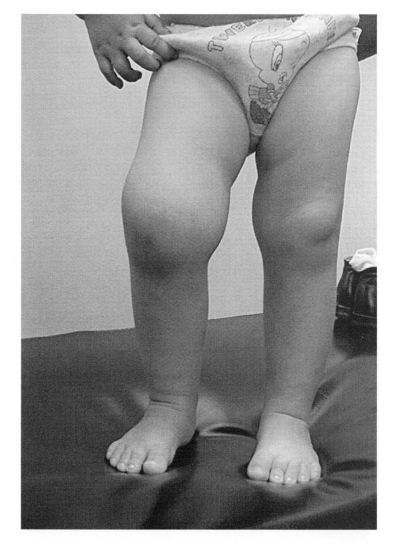

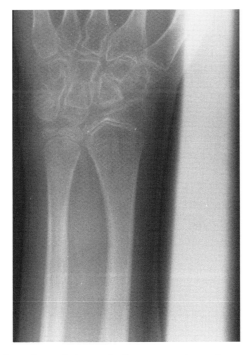

Figure 4.14. Anteroposterior radiograph demonstrating severe osteopenia and wrist joint narrowing associated with juvenile rheumatoid arthritis.

Figure 4.15. The alterations in the growth plate and the clinical appearance of Blount's disease.

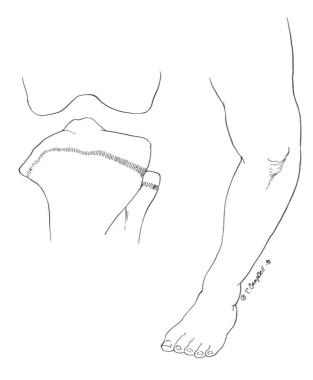

combination with a continuing physical therapy program are the basis for treatment to prevent disabling joint contractures. Bracing may prevent undesirable joint positions and provide additional support for weakened joints. Pain relief may be obtained occasionally by stabilizing painful joints. Operative synovectomy is generally reserved for those patients failing adequate medical treatment and who have persistent joint effusions with synovial thickening and joint restriction beyond a six-month period of adequate treatment.

Non-physiologic bowlegs

Nearly all cases of non-physiologic bowlegs seen in the toddler to the adolescent age group can readily be identified by radiographic evaluation of the knees. Alterations in the radiographic anatomy of the physis and the adjacent metaphysis and epiphysis are characteristic of all these conditions. A change in the texture of the bone is commonly encountered. The anatomic alterations seen on the radiograph lead one to further investigate the source of the varus. The most common conditions encountered are *infantile tibia vara* (Blount's disease) (Figures 4.15 and 4.16), rickets (nutritional, renal or Vitamin D resistant) (Figures 4.17 and 4.18), or skeletal dysplasias. Tibia vara is a disorder of unknown etiology, presenting in both infantile/ juvenile and adolescent forms (Pearl 4.5). In the infantile/ juvenile form it occurs bilaterally in over half of the cases, and most commonly presents with radiographic findings in the toddler age group. Historically, children with Blount's disease generally walk at a much earlier age than their normal counterparts (average nine to ten months walking age). It is far more common in African Americans, probably secondary to early age at walking, and the majority of children are overweight. In addition to clinical varus deformity, internal tibial torsion is always a component. The diagnosis is established by the characteristic radiographic changes. Adolescent Blount's disease is less common than infantile, is usually unilateral and has a more benign prognosis for ultimate knee formation. Treatment consists of bracing occasionally, and most often surgical correction.

Nutritional rickets or Vitamin D rickets present with the characteristic radiographic features of rickets. The diagnosis of either type is generally established in the very early toddler period and in early childhood. Nutritional rickets is currently rarely seen except in children whose diets are specifically deficient in external calcium intake or with sunlight deprivation. Vitamin D rickets is a heredity disorder (autosomal dominant), and the radiographic alterations are striking and far more severe than in nutritional rickets. In both conditions the growth plate changes are most clearly reflected in major weight bearing joints, and consist of an increase in vertical thickness of the physis, and "fraying" and "cupping" of the metaphysis. This appearance is the result of an increase in unmineralized osteoid, and an irregular pattern to the calcification process with structural weakening of the physis-metaphysis interface. "Renal" rickets or renal osteodystrophy radiographically resembles that seen in all other rachitic types. Although orthopaedic management of angular and rotational deformities in nutritional rickets may occasionally be necessary, in the form of orthotics, surgery is rarely indicated and external calcium replacement and Vitamin D generally results in healing. Cases of Vitamin D resistant rickets most commonly require metabolic drug therapy combined with orthopedic surgical realignment procedures and appropriate orthotics.

There are a considerable number of skeletal dysplasia patients that have genu varum as a component of the generalized dysplasia, and most of these patients will be short in stature. A skeletal survey to augment routine knee radiographs will generally reveal the particular

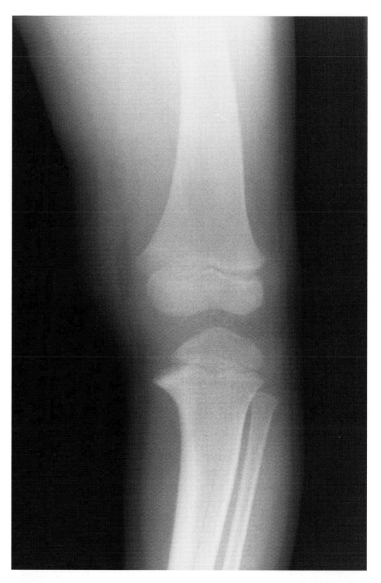

Figure 4.16. Anteroposterior radiograph showing early evidence of Blount's disease.

Pearl 4.5. Infantile Blount's disease
Severe "bow legs"
Internal tibial torsion
Radiographs
Early walking
Large body mass

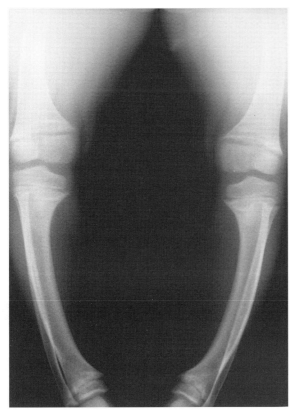

Figure 4.17. Anteroposterior radiograph showing bilateral extensive changes associated with vitamin D rickets.

Figure 4.18. Anteroposterior radiograph showing severe changes at the physis and metaphyseal regions associated with renal rickets.

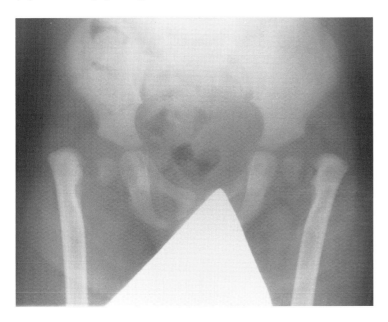

type of the skeletal dysplasia. In many of the skeletal dysplasias the affected gene has now been identified and more are increasingly being recognized.

Juvenile idiopathic scoliosis

Scoliosis is a lateral curvature of the spine combining both bending and rotation. Idiopathic scoliosis is by far the most common type of spinal deformity seen in children and adolescents. There is little concrete evidence pointing to the exact nature of the condition, although heredity has been strongly implicated. Females seem to be slightly more affected than males, and certainly have a far greater tendency toward overall progression of their curvature than do males, particularly if tall and lean.

Juvenile idiopathic scoliosis is that type of scoliosis occurring above the age of three years and prior to puberty. In contrast to infantile scoliosis, juvenile idiopathic scoliosis does not have the same propensity to spontaneously correct, and most commonly progresses. This occurs more commonly in females and many left thoracic curves are encountered. The diagnosis of idiopathic juvenile scoliosis is established in the same way as for the adolescent age group. Standing observation of the forward bent spine will clearly reveal the anatomic irregularities associated with scoliosis (Figures 4.19 and 4.20). The Cobb method of curve measurement is generally utilized by measuring perpendiculars from the vertebral endplates (Figure 4.21). Five-degree differences on sequential radiographs may be considered a significant change. Children with juvenile idiopathic scoliosis often have left thoracic curves, progressive curves (right or left), abnormal hairy patches, café-au-lait spot, neurologic findings and a higher incidence of intraspinal pathology (syringomyelia, diastematomyelia). The use of MRI has been exceptionally successful in identifying intraspinal lesions.

Although clearly some juvenile curves will remain stationary, the majority are believed to progress. Curves beyond 20 degrees in measurement with substantial clinical deformity will often require treatment (bracing) because of the length of time available for growth and the potential for progression. Generally speaking, juvenile curves are more flexible than adolescent curves, and bracing can commonly accomplish prevention of progression if compliance is adequate. Surgical treatment of scoliosis in this age group is generally reserved for failures of brace treatment or curves exceeding 40–45 degrees in dimension. Primary care physicians should be familiar with the clinical findings of scoliosis and evaluate the magnitude of the curves by appropriate radiographic means. School screening programs have produced a large number of children with curves of 10 degrees or less and many of these curves can be adequately followed by primary care physicians after appropriate instruction. It is suggested that patients with curves above these dimensions, with clinical deformity, have supplementary orthopedic consultation.

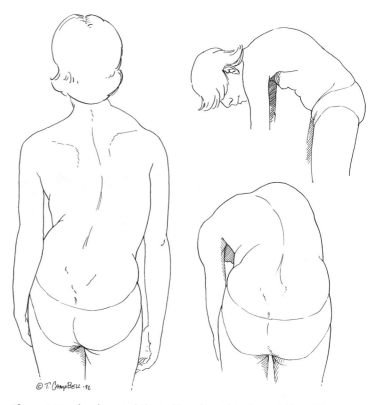

Figure 4.19. The characteristic positive physical findings of idiopathic scoliosis and positions of examination.

Popliteal cysts (ganglions)

Popliteal cysts are soft tissue masses that appear in the posterior aspect of the knee, usually in the area of the medial popliteal space. They are filled with a gelatinous fluid that commonly transilluminates. The cysts are seen most commonly in boys, and are most commonly unilateral. These cysts are herniations or "outpouchings" of the joint itself. The vast majority of the cysts seem to arise from a space between the medial head of the gastrocnemius and the semitendinosis tendon (Figure 4.22). The cysts are clearly benign and have a histologic constitution resembling that of a ganglion cyst. Baker described the lesions in 1887, giving rise to the eponym of Baker's cyst.

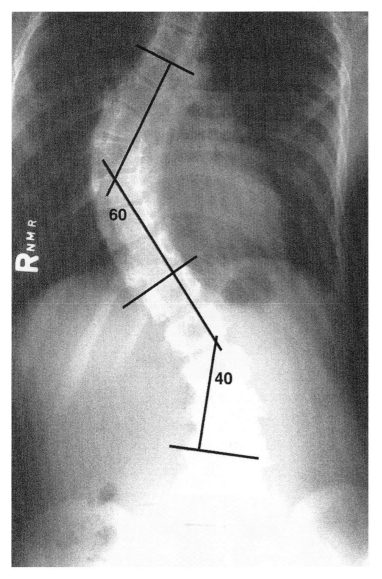

Figure 4.20. Anteroposterior radiograph of the thoracolumbar spine showing a thoracolumbar scoliosis.

Typically the lesions will enlarge as the child stands and is on his feet most of the day; most will recede by morning, as a result of the communication with the knee joint. Pain is seen only occasionally and stiffness is rarely ever seen. Radiographs generally disclose soft tissue swelling. Arthrography and computed tomography scanning are usually superfluous. Differential diagnosis includes subcutaneous lipomas, popliteal aneurysms, and benign and malignant tumors. All of these should be readily differentiated by radiographic texture, abnormal pulsation, computed tomography (CT) scanning or MRI if the cyst lies in an unusual location. After many years of surgical extirpation, with very frequent recurrences, sanity has begun to prevail, and recognition of the natural history of the disease is now being well appreciated. The vast majority of cysts will either recede in size or disappear within a two- to three-year period after clinical presentation or almost always by puberty. It is to be remembered that ganglions most commonly occur on the dorsal or volar aspects of the wrist and often communicate with the joint. In the absence of clinical symptoms, all cysts should be observed periodically and surgery should be avoided. Operations are generally reserved for those rare children who are suffering from significant pain and whose cysts persist until puberty.

Spastic torticollis

In addition to the far more common congenital muscular torticollis, there is a type of torticollis or "wryneck" that appears in the toddler to adolescent age group that is associated with either inflammatory conditions in the cervical region, traumatic lesions, tumors or neurogenic disorders. The obvious implication is that the source of the "wryneck" is secondary to some other medical condition apart from the sternocleidomastoid muscle.

One of the more common reasons for a spastic torticollis is atlantoaxial rotary "subluxation." The children present with a painful torticollis after a traumatic episode such as occurs during wrestling, tumbling or a fall. Typically the children "splint" and resist any attempts to rotate the head or the neck. The term *rotary displacement* is probably more appropriate inasmuch as it is uncommon to document any true radiographic subluxation of the atlantoaxial joint. On rare occasion CT evidence of rotary displacement may be visualized. Fortunately the condition resolves almost invariably and spontaneously, with or without treatment (physical therapy, traction, heat).

Spastic torticollis is also occasionally seen following upper respiratory infections, in association with cervical adenitis. Presumably the inflamed lymph nodes irritate the sternocleidomastoid and the anterior cervical "strap" muscles, producing the torticollis. Diagnosis is established by identifying the primary infection and treatment by the primary care physician generally results in resolution of the torticollis.

Spinal cord tumors and cerebellar tumors occasionally can produce a spastic torticollis. An adequate neurologic evaluation is mandatory and a part of evaluating all acquired cases of torticollis. Symptomatic treatment is generally used for spastic torticollis in the form of heat, massage, and intermittent cervical traction, providing there is no evidence of true cervical vertebral instability. Resolution is generally abrupt in inflammatory and atlantoaxial rotary displacements. Occasional symptoms may be encountered up to four to six weeks after the initial episode. Neurogenic torticollis demands neurologic/ neurosurgical intervention.

Subluxation of the radial head

"Pulled elbow" is most commonly seen in children between one and five years of age. It occurs following an injury sustained in which the child's forearm or hand is being held and the child attempts to fall away, or is lifted from

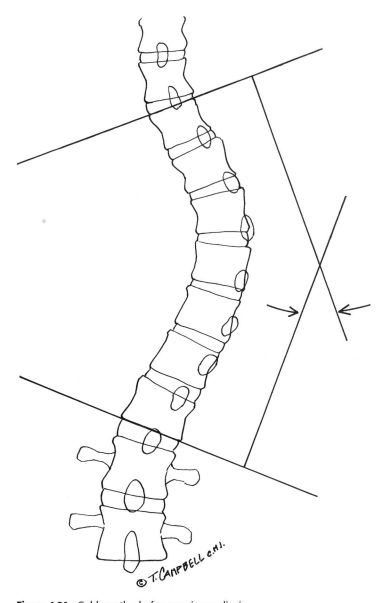

Figure 4.21. Cobb method of measuring scoliosis.

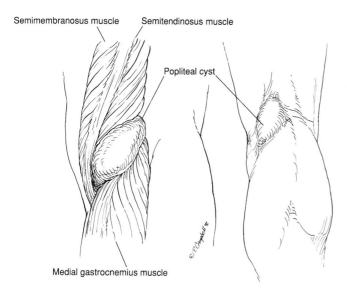

Figure 4.22. The characteristic location of a popliteal cyst between semitendinosus and gastrocnemius muscles.

Figure 4.23. The mechanism of production of subluxation of the radial head, and the characteristic position of the upper extremity at presentation.

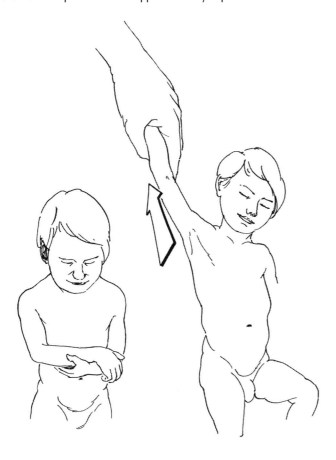

the ground by the hands. It is not produced by a fall on the outstretched hand or arm. The children tend to carry the forearm in a "lame" position of forearm pronation, and elbow flexion supported by the other hand (Figure 4.23). Supination of the forearm or pressure over the radial head increases the discomfort.

True subluxation or dislocation of the radial head from its position against the capitellum has never been demonstrated radiographically or pathologically. The condition occurs when longitudinal traction is applied to the forearm with the arm extended and the forearm pronated. It is believed that a portion of the annular ligament becomes interposed between the radial head and capitellum and then dislodges when the forearm is supinated in slight elbow flexion.

When painful, the elbow is slightly flexed and the forearm held in pronation. Reduction is achieved by supination of the forearm. A palpable and sometimes audible "click" often accompanies the immediate relief of pain.

Regardless of the exact anatomic abnormality, the condition in nearly all cases will resolve as the child reaches the end of the first decade of life. In roughly 20 percent of the cases, recurrences will be encountered, although treatment of the individual event is identical. Initial treatment generally consists of a simple reduction, sling, posterior splint, or occasional long arm cast for a brief period ranging from two to three days to two weeks. There are no indications for operative intervention. Parents experiencing repeat "subluxation" should be instructed on the reduction maneuver of supination of the forearm. Persistent discomfort following reduction may on occasion necessitate a longer period of immobilization.

Muscular dystrophies

Although there are several muscular dystrophies in childhood, three types are seen with some degree of regularity: progressive muscular dystrophy; limb-girdle dystrophy; and facio-scapulo-humeral dystrophy. By far the most prevalent form of dystrophy seen in clinical practice is the sex-linked progressive dystrophy of the Duchenne type. The disease is produced by an abnormality in the gene for the production of dystrophin. Absence or marked reduction of dystrophin results in destabilization of the muscle cell membrane which allows creatine kinase to leak into the serum with progressive loss of muscle mass and replacement by fibro-fatty tissue. This disease occurs in males, and a positive family history is frequently obtained. Initially there is symmetrical weakness of the pelvic girdle muscles followed later by generalized progressive weakness in the area of the shoulder girdle and eventually even progressing distally. Pseudohypertrophy of the calf is characteristic, but not purely diagnostic. Cardiac involvement is nearly always present, and generally death occurs from cardiopulmonary failure prior to 20 years of age. It is common in reviewing the history to uncover a delay in developmental milestones, and in fact most children will not achieve ambulation until between 18 and 24 months of age.

Commonly a history of falling easily, difficulty climbing stairs and difficulty jumping or running is obtained. Involvement of the hip extensor muscles produces a flexion deformity at the hips and a lumbar lordosis. The foot and ankle are held in equinus as a result of gastrocnemius contracture. Involvement of the hip abductors results in a "waddling" type of wide base gait. Gower's sign is commonly elicited early in the disease (Figure 4.24). This maneuver generally reflects the degree of quadriceps weakness and the inability to straighten the knee, forcing the child to literally crawl up his legs with his hands, pressing first on the knees and then the thighs to gain an erect posture.

Clinical diagnosis is established by assessing the abnormal gait, examining for specific areas of muscle weakness, the presence of a normal

Figure 4.24. The characteristic positions of Gowers sign.

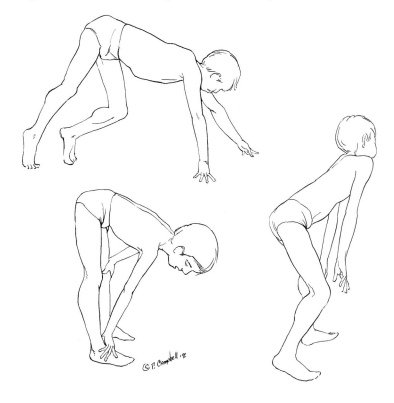

neurologic sensory examination, but diminished or absent biceps and knee jerks. Eventually all patients will become wheelchair bound, at which point scoliosis generally progresses, if already present, or develops if not present. The progression of the scoliosis is often severe enough to require surgical spinal stabilization. Average intelligence quotients for these patients have been estimated to be in the range of 80 to 90. Laboratory examination can be of considerable help in diagnosis and DNA testing is currently available. The creatine kinase level is generally increased 200–400 times normal values and reflects the extent of skeletal muscle damage. Muscle biopsy is one of the most important diagnostic studies and generally reveals degeneration of the muscle fibers and loss of muscle fibers, with variation in fiber size and a marked proliferation of fibro-fatty connective tissue (Pearl 4.6). Western bloc analysis of digested muscle tissue demonstrates reduced or absent dystrophin in affected individuals.

A milder form of muscular dystrophy, termed Becker dystrophy, has been identified, with an onset generally between 8 and 12 years of age. Ambulation is commonly maintained until the latter part of the second decade or even into the twenties and thirties. Cardiac involvement is uncommon and probably accounts for the continuing ambulatory status.

Far less commonly encountered is limb-girdle dystrophy, an autosomal recessive dystrophy. The diagnosis is generally not established until the second or third decade. It is a slowly progressive disease primarily involving the pelvic and shoulder girdles, with rare pseudohypertrophy in the calf. Cardiac involvement and intellectual impairment are uncommon. It is generally differentiated from pseudohypertrophic muscular dystrophy by the late onset, the more benign pattern, and only slight elevation of the creatine kinase level. Patients generally live into the forty to fifty year range.

Another uncommon form of muscular dystrophy seen in the later part of the first and second decade is facio-scapulo-humeral

---

Pearl 4.6. Diagnostic features of Duchenne muscular dystrophy

Clinical picture
↑Creatine kinase
Muscle biopsy
↓Dystrophin

dystrophy, an autosomal dominant disease. Cardiac involvement and intellectual impairment are generally absent. Characteristically the muscles of the shoulder girdle and face are affected, and it is a slowly progressive disorder. Clinical findings include muscle weakness, inability to close the eyes tightly, "pouting" of the lips, and absent facial wrinkles. The muscles of the shoulder girdle are involved. Diagnosis is generally established by the manual muscle test. Muscle biopsy demonstrates a dystrophic type pattern with very large muscle fibers and an inflammatory response. Interestingly the creatine kinase levels are usually within normal limits. Prognosis for longevity is often satisfactory. The role of the physician clearly rests at the level of diagnosis. An awareness of developmental delays and maturation should alert one to formally examine for any areas of muscle weakness. Once the diagnosis has been established, the needs of the patient are directed to the cardio-respiratory status combined with appropriate orthopedic management and physical therapy. Orthopaedic procedures of the spine, hip, knees and ankle level may occasionally delay the transit into a wheelchair and may also improve the quality of life, particularly in regard to the management of scoliosis by early spinal stabilization of progressive scoliosis. Recent use of corticosteroids has shown promise but long-term evaluation remains necessary.

Köhler's disease

Köhler's disease is a nutritional disorder of the tarsal navicular that results in an avascular necrosis. It is thought to occur as a consequence of cumulative minor traumata. It nearly always makes its appearance between the age of three and seven years, and is somewhat more common in males. The child presents with an antalgic limp with pain localized on compression in the area of the

(a)

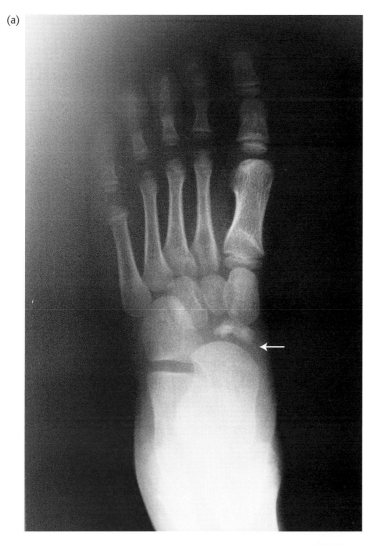

(b)

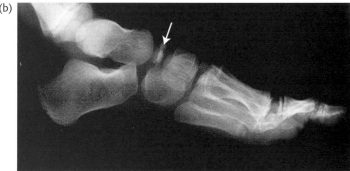

Figure 4.25. (a) Anteroposterior radiograph showing the osseous changes of the tarsal navicular seen in Köhler's disease. (b) Lateral radiograph showing the characteristic fragmentation and sclerosis and change in shape seen in Köhler's disease.

tarsal navicular. Occasionally some localized swelling is recognized.

The diagnosis is established by a combination of symptomatology coupled with a radiographically fragmented, irregularly dense appearance to the tarsal navicular (Figures 4.25a, b). The tarsal navicular does not begin to ossify until roughly age three and often may be irregular and fragmented as a normal variation in its ensuing ossification pattern. The diagnosis of Köhler's disease should be established only when there is a combination of radiographic findings and localized symptomatology. Treatment consists of short-term casting and perhaps brief periods of diminished weight bearing. Orthotics have also been helpful on occasion. The prognosis is uniformly excellent with symptomatology disappearing generally within several months after its appearance. Orthopedic referral is appropriate.

Discoid meniscus

Discoid meniscus is usually seen between one and eight years of age although occasional cases have been seen under one year of age. A child with a discoid meniscus commonly will present with a complaint of a "clunk" or a "clicking" sensation in the knee with or without discomfort. Occasionally "falling" or reluctance to move the knee through a range of motion is observed. Symptoms are almost always related to activities. On examination, a characteristic "clunk" or "snap" is perceived on moving the knee through a range of flexion and extension. The clinical findings are most commonly directed to the lateral compartment of the knee and the lateral joint line.

The basic pathoanatomy is the presence of a discoid-shaped meniscus rather than the normal semilunar shape usually present in the lateral compartment of the knee joint (Figure 4.26). Occasionally a discoid meniscus can appear on the medial side, but only very rarely. The thickened mal-shaped meniscus may act as a mechanical restraint to joint motion. It may also undergo degeneration from trauma and develop a torn meniscus. Cystic changes within the meniscus have also been reported. An increased lateral joint space on plain radiography may be seen but MRI is more definitive. Treatment is designed to relieve discomfort and increase knee motion. Surgical removal (arthroscopically) of a portion or the entire discoid meniscus is indicated only if disability is present. Once the diagnosis has been established, appropriate orthopedic referral is indicated.

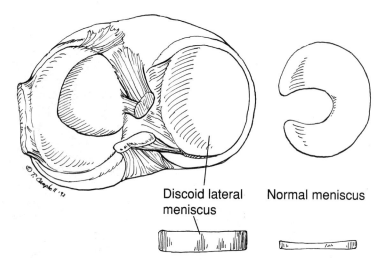

Discoid lateral meniscus

Normal meniscus

Figure 4.26. The pathoanatomy of a discoid meniscus.

Chapter 5

Adolescence and puberty

Figure 5.1. Anteroposterior radiograph demonstrating significant thoracolumbar scoliosis.

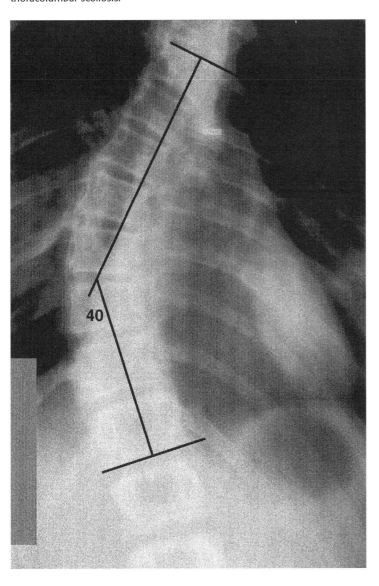

Idiopathic adolescent scoliosis

Scoliosis is a combination of spinal bending (list) and spinal rotation. Idiopathic adolescent scoliosis is the most common type of spinal deformity. Currently the diagnosis of idiopathic adolescent scoliosis encompasses those curves of 10 degrees or more. The most prevalent period for its presentation is between 10 and 15 years of age, with some variation in individuals relative to the degree of skeletal maturation. The most common curvature encountered is a right thoracic scoliosis. The next most common type of curvature is a left lumbar scoliosis, with the third most common being a thoracolumbar curve (Figure 5.1). Other curve patterns are seen far less commonly. Although the etiology is presently unknown, there is a strong hereditary pattern and a greater prevalence in females. Although school screening programs have uncovered a great number of males with the condition, reducing the ratio to roughly two to one in favor of females, the percentage of those females progressing their curvature is substantially higher, particularly tall and lean females.

Unfortunately there is no technique at present to determine which curve is going to progress, resolve or remain static. Progression has been correlated with the degree of skeletal maturation, the location of the curve, and the curve magnitude. In general, spinal curvatures initially seen in late adolescence do not progress beyond skeletal maturation, if the curvature is less than a 30-degree magnitude.

Thoracic curvatures greater than thirty degrees have been shown to progress in some cases. From the primary care standpoint, patients with thoracic curvatures between 40 and 45 degrees or greater are generally considered surgical candidates for spinal fusion and instrumentation. Cardiopulmonary decompensation is usually not encountered until thoracic curves reach 50–60 degrees. Nearly 90 to 95 percent of all curvatures seen by physicians will be below 40 degrees, with the vast majority below 20 degrees. Patients with thoracic curvatures between 20 and 40 degrees, with cosmetic deformity, form the primary clinical nucleus for which spinal bracing (orthotics) has been used. Decision-making before embarking on the use of bracing is dependent on the magnitude of the curvature, the magnitude of clinical deformity, the location of the curve and the degree of skeletal maturation. Curves 10 degrees or less can be appropriately followed at intervals by a primary care physician until skeletal maturation is reached.

The clinical findings of a spinal curvature are readily detected in a very brief examination (Figure 5.2). Those findings most commonly noted are asymmetry of the height of the shoulder, as reflected by the trapezial slope, asymmetry of the inferior and medial border of the scapula when standing erect, asymmetry of the lumbar creases, prominent rib bulge on 90 degree forward bending, or a prominent lumbar muscular bulge. Furthermore, when standing erect a plumb line dropped from the seventh cervical spinous process should rest completely within the gluteal crease. Curves secondary to limb length inequality will generally show no evidence of spinal rotation or vertebral deformation. The diagnosis is easily established, and after assessing the magnitude of the curvature, a determination will be required as to the need for any further specialty care.

Figure 5.2. The examination position and clinical findings of scoliosis and Scheuermann's disease.

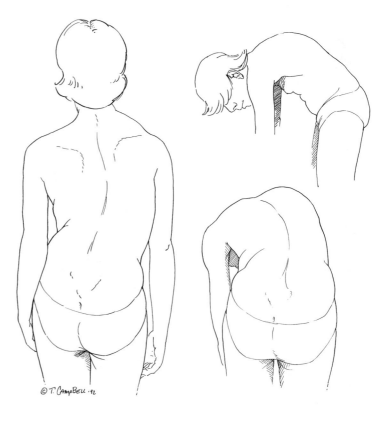

Scheuermann's disease

The second most common type of spinal deformity seen by physicians is *adolescent roundback,* or Scheuermann's disease. The condition results in a "roundback" or "humpback" deformity, is best visualized from the side on lateral bending, is seen equally in males and females, and generally is found in patients between 12 and 16 years of age. Commonly there is a hereditary pattern to its presentation but the exact mode of transmission is unknown. The vast majority of cases of Scheuermann's disease are located in the thoracic spine region, with roughly one-fourth or less occurring in the lumbar region.

At least half of the patients so affected will present with back pain as a significant part of their symptomatology. Although the exact etiology is continuously debated, it is clear that there is a disorder of growth of the ring epiphyses of the thoracic and lumbar vertebrae. The vertebrae end plates are often "irregular" and "frayed," particularly anteriorly, and distortion is evident in the subchondral bone adjacent to the "limbic" (ring) epiphysis (Figure 5.3). This disproportionate reduction in anterior to posterior vertebral height likely reflects asymmetrical compression. The sequela of this physeal abnormality is an architectural alteration in the shape of the vertebra, progressing from a rectangular shape to more of a "trapezoidal" or "wedge" shape. If this disorder affects the thoracic spine, the deformity produced is one of kyphosis or kyphoscoliosis. If the deformity affects the lumbar spine there will commonly be straightening of the lumbar spine or a localized lumbar kyphosis. Tight hamstrings are commonly detected on forward bending. A substantial number of patients with Scheuermann's disease have an associated spondylolysis. The pain related by the patient may be mechanical in nature and associated with activities or may occur at rest, occasionally

Figure 5.3. Lateral radiograph demonstrating "wedging" and characteristic vertebral changes seen in Scheuermann's disease.

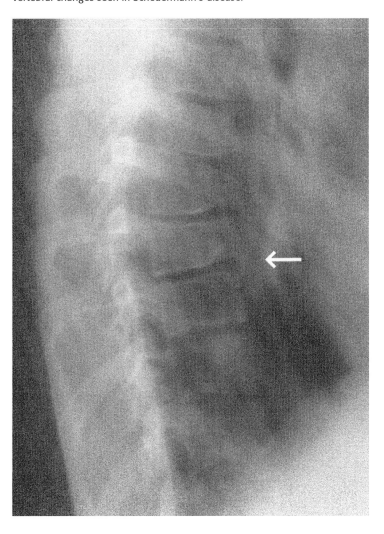

occurring at night, and may be more characteristic of an inflammatory type of pain.

Standard conservative regimens (heat, rest, massage, and anti-inflammatory medication) usually will ameliorate the symptoms, although occasionally disparaging symptoms may necessitate spinal orthotics. By the conclusion of skeletal maturation, the pain has almost always subsided, leaving whatever degree of spinal deformity remaining.

The primary disorder to be differentiated by physicians will be "postural" kyphosis. Children and adolescents presenting with "postural" kyphosis will have a "flexible" spine and can change their degree of kyphosis (deformity) simply by positioning. Prone lateral radiographs will show a distinct reduction in the degree of kyphosis. Patients with Scheuermann's disease will maintain their thoracic deformity, whether standing radiographs or supine or prone radiographs are taken. Furthermore, "postural" kyphosis is not accompanied by anatomic changes within the vertebrae. In the thoracic region, normal degrees of kyphosis have been estimated to measure as high as 50 degrees without anatomic vertebral wedging. Patients with greater than 50 degrees of kyphosis associated with characteristic signs of vertebral "wedging" and irregularities of the growth plate demonstrate findings compatible with Scheuermann's disease. Disc space irregularity and Schmorl's nodes are common. Generally three to five vertebrae are involved. Magnetic resonance imaging (MRI) may be necessary in cases with accompanying neurologic defects. The natural history of Scheuermann's disease is for slow progression to occur during the adolescent growing years, and to stabilize when skeletal maturation approaches. Pulmonary compromise rarely occurs in patients with less than 60 degrees of curvature.

Postural exercises, although usually prescribed, have never been shown to provide any significant improvement in the degree of kyphosis. Spinal orthotics are generally instituted for curves measuring below

60 degrees with definite radiographic evidence of Scheuermann's disease and can be effective although orthotic compliance is difficult to document, as with scoliosis. Occasionally patients experiencing chronic unremitting pain, who are skeletally mature, and whose curves are 60 degrees or more may warrant surgical stabilization by fusion and instrumentation. From the standpoint of the primary care physician, it is important to be aware of this condition and to establish the correct diagnosis. Appropriate orthopedic referral should be recommended.

Backache and disc disease

Traditionally, it has been taught that children and adolescents rarely experience back pain and when they do, significant underlying pathology is often present and aggressive investigation is necessary to determine the cause. More recently, however, it has been recognized that back pain is far more common, at least in adolescents, than previously appreciated. Indeed the numbers appear quite similar to those in adults; about 80 percent will have pain that resolves in roughly six weeks and will demonstrate no clear pathologic diagnosis. Accordingly, aggressive investigation into etiology should be undertaken only in selective cases to avoid "medicalizing" transient problems, unnecessarily disturbing parents, identifying radiographic false positives, and unnecessary radiation. It is incumbent on the physician to recognize those children who require a more intense evaluation based upon certain key indicators. A careful history and physical examination are imperative. (1) Pain which does not respond to simple conservative measures (periodic bed rest, temporary activity restriction, physical therapy, and anti-inflammatories) within six weeks. (2) Pain which is "non-mechanical" in nature; pain that is worse at night or unrelieved by unloading the spine. (3) Pain that is associated with a significant trauma. (4) Pain that is associated with systemic signs of infection. (5) Pain that is associated with neurologic (motor, sensory, reflex, or bladder) abnormality. As always, a good history and physical examination will rarely mislead the physician.

Without question, the most common source of back pain in the adolescent is trauma. In adolescents, mechanical soft tissue strains and bony injury exceed all other causes of back pain combined. Because of the resiliency of the tissues in an adolescent, musculo-ligamentous sprains are far more common than bony injuries. This is directly related to the greater degree of elasticity of the growing spine. There is nothing peculiar to the management of these conditions in childhood as compared with an adult. The remarkable capacity of children to recuperate rather than succumb makes prolonged disability unusual. Spondylolisthesis is probably the next most frequent cause of back pain and is discussed in a later section.

Intervertebral disc disease in children is an uncommon cause of back pain but can occur particularly in adolescents. Although the disc can and does degenerate, protrude, sequestrate, and impinge on nerve roots, it does so uncommonly compared with the frequency seen in middle aged adults (Figure 5.4). On closer scrutiny there seems to be a high incidence of other family members with manifest degenerative disc disease. The history of pre-existent back trauma is much more readily obtained in children than in adults. There is no sex predilection. Nearly all cases are seen in the second decade of life. Involvement of the L5–S1 interspace appears to be the most frequent location for presentation. Magnetic resonance imaging when indicated is the diagnostic test of choice.

The indications for conservative and surgical treatment are nearly identical to the adult. It is the rather consistent impression of surgeons caring for this disorder in adolescents that the long-term results of surgical treatment, regardless of type, do not parallel those of the adult, and are routinely poorer. This may in part be due to the fact that these youngsters

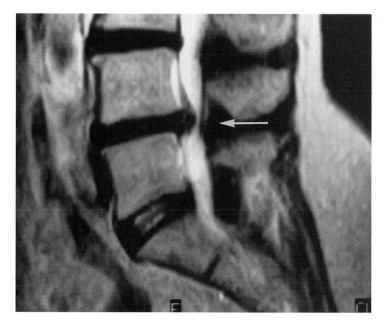

Figure 5.4. Magnetic resonance imaging demonstrating intervertebral disc protrusion.

have already demonstrated a genetic weakness within the disc itself, and that they will show other signs of difficulty at other levels later in life. Conservative treatment with physical therapy modalities, non-steroid anti-inflammatories and rest commonly results in resolution of symptoms in 80 to 90 percent of patients within six weeks.

Disc space infection in children may occur in this age group but is quite uncommon when compared with the first decade of life. Back pain occurring in concert with idiopathic adolescent scoliosis is a common complaint when carefully scrutinized. Roughly half of the patients with idiopathic adolescent scoliosis will have intermittent complaints of aching pain but rarely of sufficient nature to require either urgent medical care or hospitalization. The source of these symptoms is unclear but they are generally quite responsive to conservative methods.

Tumors are the source of pain in less than five percent of children and adolescents with pain that persists despite appropriate conservative care. Focal, "boring," deep pain, which often is worse at night, should raise suspicion. Systemic frailty is often noted. Evaluation should include anterior–posterior and lateral radiographs of the involved region, with bone scan or MRI if suspicion is high. Malignant tumors such as osteosarcoma, neuroblastoma or Ewing's sarcoma can present with spine pain often associated with bony destruction. Benign tumors such as hemangiomas, aneurysmal bone cysts, and osteoblastomas can also cause pain from cortical intraosseous pressure or pathologic fracture. Osteoid osteomas or osteoblastomas generally produce inflammatory-like pain. Again, careful, thorough, and high quality physical evaluation should provide an early diagnosis and prompt referral is recommended.

An uncommon cause of back pain in adolescents, but one with serious ramifications is ankylosing spondylitis (Marie–Strumpell arthritis). Although ankylosing spondylitis is generally diagnosed during the late second and third decades of life, in retrospect, many patients have developed symptoms during adolescence. Backache and stiffness are the two characteristic complaints. The backache is most frequently nocturnal, dull and nagging in nature, and presents at rest although occasionally it can be mechanical in nature. Stiffness is quite common and generally encountered on arising early in the morning or after arising from recumbency. Cervical, dorsal, or lumbar involvement at the onset are the usual modes of presentation although eventually nearly all the spinal areas are involved, particularly the sacroiliac joints. Roughly 50 percent of the time peripheral joints are affected, but rarely to the extent seen in the full-blown adult polyarticular rheumatoid arthritis. Elevated sedimentation rates and HLAW B27 may be helpful in diagnosis.

It is difficult to overlook the many similarities to rheumatoid arthritis, including the pathologic process itself. Etiology is still obscure but it probably should be classified as a distinct disorder by itself with a relatively good life prognosis. Early cases of demise from aortic insufficiency, amyloidosis, and subluxation of the atlantoaxial articulation have been recorded but are still the exception. The disease has a strong hereditary background, although the exact mode of transmission is unclear. Ankylosing spondylitis is seen nearly 10 times more commonly in males. The disease throughout the spine and sacroiliac joints tends to progress with time toward ankylosis of all spinal joints, with a characteristic calcification of the periarticular structures commonly seen on radiographs. There is a marked cervical lordosis and an increasing thoracic kyphosis. The ensuing rapid progression of the kyphosis presents a disheartening situation in merely keeping abreast of the spinal deformity. Eventually spinal fixation occurs and the pain comes under control. Roughly three-quarters of all patients will be independently supporting themselves later so that all efforts to prevent progression seem worth the expenditure. Occasionally spinal surgery in the form of

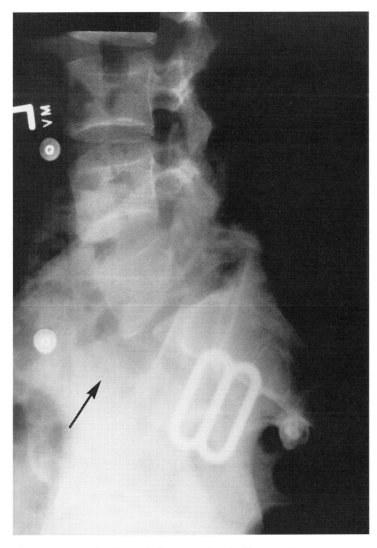

Figure 5.5. Lateral radiograph demonstrating significant L5-S1 spondylolisthesis.

osteotomy may be necessary in the thoracolumbar and cervical regions. Certainly this condition should be considered in adolescents with back pain that is not purely mechanical in nature, and particularly in those with episodes of recurrence and spinal stiffness.

Spondylolisthesis

Forward slipping of one vertebra on another (spondylolisthesis), has been recognized as a cause of back disability in adolescence for over 200 years. *Spondylolysis* is the term used to describe the defect in the pars interarticularis regardless of the extent of any slipping. Although there are five separate types of spondylolisthesis, the spondylolytic type is the most commonly encountered (Figure 5.5). The spondylolytic type of spondylolisthesis occurs in approximately two to six percent of Americans. The defect is generally recognized between four and seven years of age or older. The fifth lumbar segment is involved at least 80 percent of the time. The fourth lumbar segment is the second most commonly involved. It is generally agreed that forward slipping, if it is going to occur, will occur and progress prior to the age of 20 years and usually over a two-year period of time from the time of its presentation. Recent studies have indicated that repetitive chronic trauma is the likely cause of the defect. It appears that a stress fracture precedes the spondylolisthesis. The overall incidence of spondylolisthesis is higher in gymnasts, football linemen, wrestlers, and dancers.

There is no question that spondylolytic spondylolisthesis is a significant cause of backache in children and adolescents and often of disabling proportions. Clinically the patients will present with lumbar back pain, occasionally an exaggerated lumbar lordosis in the area of slipping, and hamstring tightness. Pain is generally elicited with forward bending and pressure on the spinous processes of L4 and L5. There may or may not be neurologic findings of sciatic stretch in the lower extremity. Clinical suspicion should prompt radiographic examination to reveal the spondylolytic defect, or true spondylolisthesis. Radionucleotide imaging currently is the most desirous means of establishing a diagnosis of spondylolysis. Computed tomography (CT) scanning can be useful in further delineating the extent of the defect and in following any potential healing of the defect in those cases of "acquired" stress fracture. Appropriate diagnosis should lead to orthopedic referral. In general, conservative back programs are used for minimal degrees of slipping. Occasionally spinal orthotics are used and surgical stabilization or reduction of the degree of the slipping may be necessary for more severe degrees of spondylolisthesis or chronic debilitating pain. Observation, at least until skeletal maturity, is recommended.

Slipped capital femoral epiphysis

Slipped capital femoral epiphysis, is a disorder of puberty characterized by slipping (movement) of the femoral head off the femoral neck. The femoral head ultimately migrates into a position of posterior–inferior displacement relative to the femoral neck. The displacement may be sudden (acute) and produce an unstable situation in which the femoral head is mobile on the femoral neck, or it may occur slowly over a period of time, and produce a stable head–neck relationship in which the head is anchored to the femoral neck, but in a displaced position (Figures 5.6 and 5.7).

Current thoughts on etiology reside with two possible hypotheses. Proponents of the mechanical theory believe that excessive body weight, seen commonly in this condition, wears out the ability of the physis to withstand the mechanical forces applied to the growth plate. By overloading, the growth plate slowly or abruptly yields to excessive body mass, resulting in slipping of the head off the femoral neck. A contrasting hypothesis suggests that

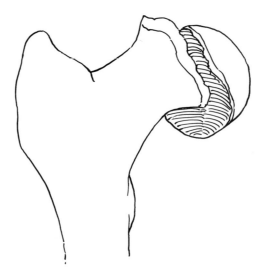

Figure 5.6. The head to neck relationship in acute slipped capital femoral epiphysis.

Figure 5.7. Lateral radiograph demonstrating bilateral slipped capital femoral epiphysis.

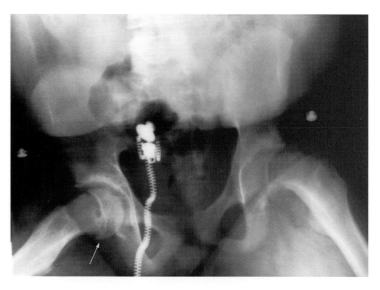

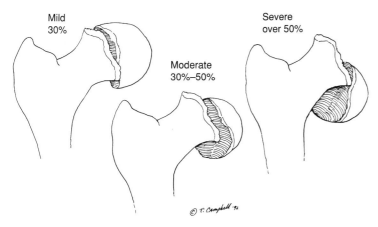

Mild
30%

Moderate
30%–50%

Severe
over 50%

© T. Campbell '92

Figure 5.8. The degrees of slipping in slipped capital femoral epiphysis compared.

the growth plate is weakened, due to a delicate imbalance between the hormones of puberty, coupled with an oblique shape to the growth plate, and excessive body mass, leading to gradual or abrupt slipping of the femoral head. This theory suggests that there is a basic hormonal imbalance at puberty that weakens the growth plate as a predilection to slipping.

Slipping usually is seen in females between 10 and 15 years of age or in males generally between 12 and 16 years of age. Males are affected slightly more often than females, in a three to two proportion. Bilateral involvement has been estimated to occur in 25 percent of the patients with a slightly higher percentage in females. Chronic slipping, where the head is anchored well to the femoral neck (stable), is seen far more commonly than acute slipping (90 percent), in which the femoral head is mobile on the femoral neck (unstable). The degree of slipping of the femoral head off the femoral neck is generally graded as to the amount of head displaced in proportion to the width of the femoral neck (Figure 5.8). Slips are generally graded as mild, with up to 30 percent displacement of the femoral head on the neck, moderate or grade two, with 30–50 percent displacement of the femoral head on the neck, and severe, with greater than 50 percent of the head displaced on the femoral neck. Histologic examination of growth plates affected by slipping have shown a general disorganization of the growth plate, with an acceleration of the chondroblast cell turnover (apoptosis), and a reduced amount and poor orientation of the collagen in the hypertrophic zone of the growth plates. In spite of these histologic abnormalities, little has been contributed to the actual discovery of the etiology, and it is still not known whether this condition is based on a purely mechanical disorder of the growth plate or a biochemical disorder. It is highly likely that the etiology is multifactorial with a preponderance of evidence favoring a "disorder" of puberty.

The clinical picture is characterized by an antalgic limp, seen in the adolescent age group, with pain generally referred along the anteromedial aspect of the thigh to the knee. The pain is accentuated by physical activity and recedes with rest. The lower extremity involved usually lies in some external rotation. The degree of limitation of range of motion clearly depends on the severity of slipping. In general, internal rotation, flexion, and abduction are limited and the degree of limitation being dependent on the magnitude of slipping. Forced accentuation of these motions is generally painful. Commonly there is shortening of the extremity, depending on how superiorly the femoral neck comes to rest in relationship to the femoral head. In cases of acute slipping (unstable), there is a profound increase in the degree of pain, the youngsters are commonly unable to walk, and severe pain is induced by any attempts at internal rotation.

Diagnosis is based on the radiographic changes commensurate with slipped capital femoral epiphysis. These include measurements of head migration from the femoral neck, physiolysis, or lytic changes adjacent to the metaphysis on the metaphyseal side of the growth plate. Physicians should always consider the possibility of this diagnosis in an adolescent patient with a painful limp. The appropriate treatment currently is surgical in all cases. Surgery involves the use of metallic internal fixation to stabilize the femoral head and prevent it from progressing (Figure 5.9) or the use of bone graft epiphyseodesis (Figure 5.10) designed to enhance the rapid closure of the growth plate, thereby preventing any further slipping. In cases in which severe deformity is already present, compensatory femoral osteotomies to change the angle of the femoral head in relation to the femoral shaft have been used to increase motion and length, and to realign the anatomy of the upper end of the femur.

There are complications associated with the basic disease as well as the treatment modalities. Avascular necrosis can be encountered in cases of acute unstable slipping regardless of treatment type; chondrolysis,

Figure 5.9. Anteroposterior radiograph demonstrating multiple metallic internal fixation used to stabilize slipped capital femoral epiphysis.

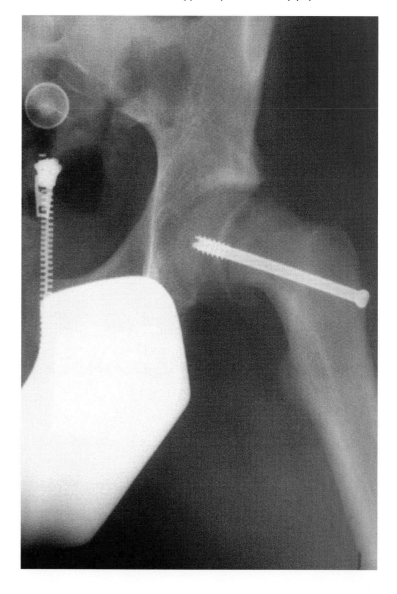

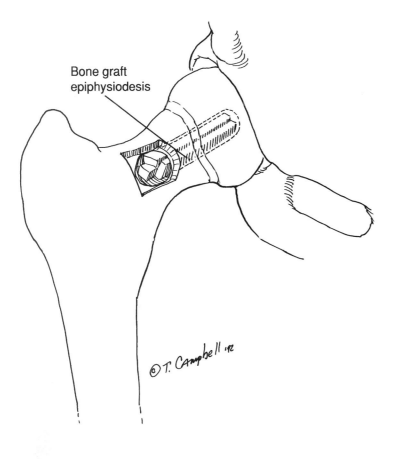

Figure 5.10. The position of bone graft in bone graft epiphyseodesis.

Figure 5.11. Anteroposterior radiograph showing metatarsus primus varus as the basic pathoanatomy of juvenile bunions.

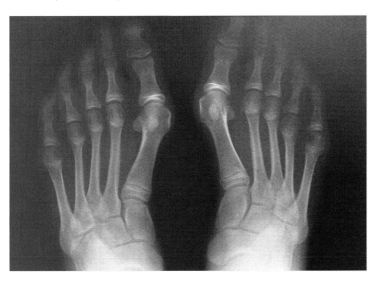

(progressive joint space narrowing) may occur in the presence of untreated slipped epiphysis, in association with metallic internal fixation and also with pin penetration.

The final common prognosis for all cases of slipped epiphysis will be determined in early middle age as to whether premature arthritis of the hip develops, or whether a normal pain-free hip will evolve. Treatment is designed to prevent further slipping, and to return the patient to a reasonably normal lifestyle during the growing years. Early recognition of this condition by physicians greatly facilitates urgent appropriate treatment, and reduces the need for reconstructive hip procedures at a later time.

Juvenile–adolescent bunions

Juvenile–adolescent bunions virtually always arise from a similar etiology. The condition of origin has been termed *metatarsus primus varus with associated bunion formation*, and this accurately describes the nature of the condition better than any other terminology. In nearly all cases there is a severe deformity (medial deviation) of the first metatarsal in relation to the second, third, fourth, and fifth metatarsals (Figure 5.11). The first metatarsal grows more and more apart from the second and more into varus. Because of the soft tissue attachments (adductor hallucis primarily) to the proximal phalanx of the great toe, the proximal and distal phalanx of the great toe deviate laterally, producing hallux valgus. The bunion itself is a "bursitis" overlying the medial portion of the head of the first metatarsal, a consequence of contact (friction) with shoe wear. However, ill-fitting shoe wear is not the primary etiologic factor in the juvenile–adolescent bunion. The primary anatomic deformity is a consequence of the metatarsus primus varus. In fact, management of the juvenile–adolescent bunion is dependent on reducing the consistently increased intermetatarsal angle. A positive family history is often encountered.

Clinically patients present for treatment at the time of adolescence, usually between 10 and 14 years of age. The first metatarsal head is prominent and there is hallux valgus present with lateral deviation of the proximal and distal phalanx of the great toe. Frequently there is a painful bursa overlying the medial portion of the first metatarsal head. Standing radiographs will consistently reveal an increased intermetatarsal angle commonly ranging between 12 and 25 degrees.

Initial management should be conservative, and is directed at altering the type of shoe wear that exacerbates the symptomatology. Patients are advised to seek whatever sort of shoe wear that will make them comfortable, and to vary the type of shoe wear until an appropriate shoe is successful. Roughly one half of all patients will fail adaptations in shoe wear, and will seek permanent alteration of the deformity. Surgical procedures are directed at removing the marked medial bony prominence of the first metatarsal, coupled with realignment procedures of the first metatarsal to reduce the metatarsus primus varus. Failure to obtain appropriate realignment of the first metatarsal will nearly always result in recurrence. Several operative options are available. The primary care physician should be aware of this condition and make appropriate orthopedic referral.

Peroneal spastic flatfoot – tarsal coalition

Peroneal spastic flatfoot is a term used to describe a stiff, painful foot, which appears to have accompanying flattening of the longitudinal arch. The condition is accompanied by "spasm" of the peroneal tendons. The etiology of this condition is diverse, and may occur in association with fractures of the hindfoot, rheumatoid arthritis,

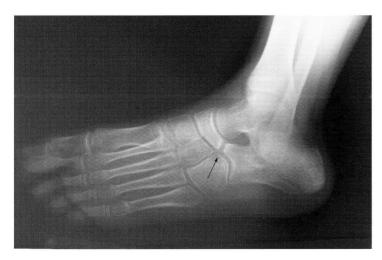

Figure 5.12. Oblique radiograph clearly demonstrating calcaneal navicular bar (tarsal coalition).

Figure 5.13. Computed tomography image demonstrating medial facet talocalcaneal coalition.

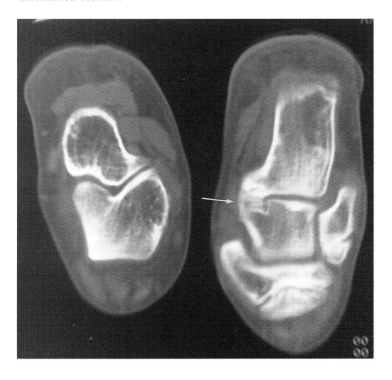

or bony fusion of the bones of the hindfoot (tarsal coalition). Without question, the vast majority of cases seen are associated with tarsal coalitions. It is likely that the condition occurs in less than one percent of the population, and is nearly always seen at the time of adolescence and puberty. There is no specific sex predilection, and no hereditary background. The most common coalition is that between the calcaneus and the navicular (Figure 5.12), although subtalar coalitions are nearly as common (Figure 5.13). The actual coalition may be fibrous, cartilaginous, or osseous. Bilaterality occurs in at least one-third of the cases.

Clinically the condition presents as a painful foot in an adolescent accompanied by rigidity of the hindfoot and peroneal "spasm" in response to attempts to invert the foot. The presence of a painful stiff foot in the adolescent age range should immediately alert the physician to the possibility of a tarsal coalition. The diagnosis is then established by appropriate radiographic examination of the hindfoot to include anteroposterior, lateral and oblique radiographs. If clinical suspicion is not satisfied, then a CT scan of the hindfoot is indicated, and is probably the most accurate means of determining the presence or absence of a hindfoot coalition. Occasionally MRI may be necessary to delineate fibrous coalitions.

Although conservative treatment in the form of casting and orthotics is occasionally successful, the vast majority of patients will become recalcitrant, and continue with symptomatology, warranting surgical intervention. Current surgical management includes the use of operative procedures designed to separate the coalition by resection of the bar, or fusion of the joints involved (triple or subtalar arthrodesis). Surgical treatment has been successful in roughly 90 percent of all cases. The primary physician's role is to be cognizant of the clinical presentation and to institute appropriate orthopedic referral.

Recurrent subluxation (dislocation) of the patella

Recurrent subluxation, or dislocation of the patella, is a condition most commonly seen in adolescents and teenagers, most commonly occurs in females, with a definite familial background. A congenital form is recognized and is most commonly associated with other disorders or syndromes (Down syndrome, skeletal dysplasias, Ehlers–Danlos syndrome, and arthrogryposis). When seen in its most common form it is nearly always associated with generalized ligamentous laxity. In association with ligamentous laxity there is evidence of contracture of the lateral soft tissue supports of the patella, particularly the lateral retinaculum and capsule and vastus lateralis tendon insertion. Children in this age group often will have a significant degree of genu valgum, external tibial torsion and/ or a significant amount of internal femoral torsion.

The most common presenting symptoms are that of episodes of "giving way" with pain in the knee and occasional "popping." The symptoms are generally encountered when the knee is brought into the last thirty to forty degrees of full extension. There may be accompanying symptoms of "grating." In its fullest form the patella may dislocate as the knee comes into full extension. The source of these symptoms is believed to be due to the malalignment of the patella within the femoral intercondylar groove, and most likely is related to a roughened area on the patella "rubbing" onto the synovial surface. Dislocation merely represents a more advanced stage of subluxation.

The diagnosis is established by examining the "tracking" of the patella as the knee is brought from full flexion into full extension. Commonly a "figure four" sign is seen, or a "Q" sign, which relates to the movement of the patella within the intercondylar groove as the knee is brought into full extension (Figure 5.14). In full extension it is usually

Figure 5.14. Abnormal patellar "tracking" seen during knee extension in chronic patellar subluxation.

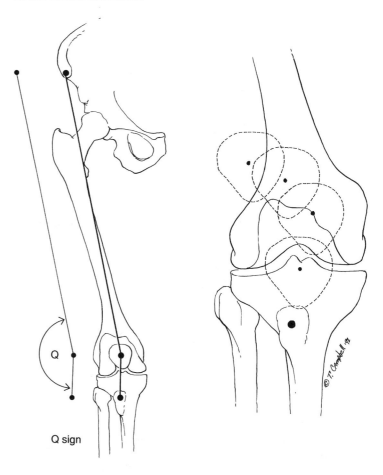

Q sign

possible to displace the patella laterally with very little pressure (light thumb pressure). Provocative pressure on the patella in an attempt to sublux the patella laterally will often elicit "guarding" or apprehension on the patient's behalf. Guarding is commonly observed with the knee at 20–30 degrees of flexion. Not uncommonly, there will be tenderness over the medial capsule and retinaculum on direct pressure. Although radiographs may be occasionally helpful in discerning the relative degree of formation of the lateral condyle and the position of the patella within the groove, the diagnosis is established on a clinical basis.

Long-term disability encountered with this condition relates to the degree of subluxation and dislocations and the length of time the dislocations have been occurring. Chronic dislocations will likely result in wear and tear changes on the undersurface of the patella as well as on the lateral femoral condyle, and can indeed precipitate premature patellofemoral arthritis. An awareness of the diagnostic features will facilitate appropriate orthopedic referral by the primary care physician. Although treatment is often conservative, with exercises to maintain quadriceps strength, and occasional bracing to inhibit lateral subluxation, a number of youngsters will fail conservative care and will require surgical realignment. A variety of surgical realignment approaches are available, with satisfactory results to be anticipated in the majority of cases if performed prior to the development of patellofemoral arthritis.

Pain syndromes of adolescence

Patellofemoral pain syndrome

Traditionally patellofemoral pain syndrome had been termed *chondromalacia patella* and probably accounts for the greatest number of all cases of knee pain seen in adolescents. The reason for the terminology change relates to the fact that most cases of the patellofemoral pain syndrome do not show pathologic evidence of true chondromalacia of the patella, by either gross anatomic or histologic changes. Characteristically, it is seen more commonly in females although it is often seen in males. The pain is always of a mechanical nature, commonly occurs with activity, and particularly is exacerbated by traveling up and down stairs. Bike riding, running, jumping, and knee squats will frequently reproduce the symptoms. Pain is generally associated with episodes of "giving way." On closer scrutiny of these symptoms, it can be determined that the "giving way" tends to occur in concert with the pain, although the knee rarely ever "collapses" and rarely does the patient ever fall to the ground. Occasional episodes of swelling (joint effusion) may occur.

This condition is quite commonly seen in association with recurrent subluxation or dislocation of the patella, and these conditions must be differentiated from the more commonly seen patellofemoral pain syndrome. The natural history of this syndrome is important. In contrast to the anatomic malalignment seen in recurrent subluxation and dislocation, this condition tends to spontaneously resolve in the vast majority of patients. It has been estimated that nearly 90 percent of all cases will resolve by the end of the second to third decade. Probably less than 10 percent of patients develop prolonged disabling symptoms requiring surgical treatment.

It has been found from experiences with open arthrotomy and arthroscopic examination that true chondromalacia of the patella is generally not part of this pathologic process. Although joint effusion may be noted on physical examination, with pain on compression of the patella laterally, and tenderness over the medial retinaculum, the most important clinical finding is provocative reproduction of the pain, by "trapping" the patella in the femoral groove against a forced contraction of the quadriceps (Figure 5.15). As

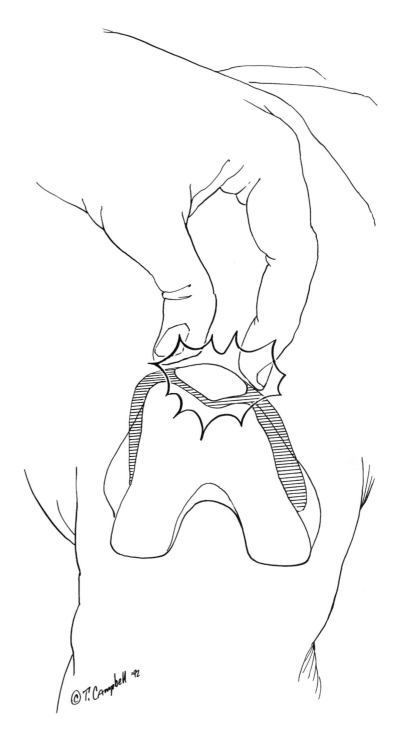

Figure 5.15. Compression of the patella in the intercondylar groove producing the characteristic pain.

the patient begins to fully contract the quadriceps, the patella is compressed against the synovial lining with reproduction of typical pain. Not uncommonly a sensation of "grating" will also be perceived. There are no radiographic features diagnostic of the condition, but radiographs should be taken to differentiate other causes of knee pain.

Treatment is clearly conservative, consisting of a combination of ice, heat, short-arc quadriceps exercises, nonsteroidal anti-inflammatory pain medication, and occasionally stretching exercises of the hamstrings and gastrocnemius muscles to reduce the tension on the patellofemoral articulation. Cases recalcitrant to conservative treatment may occasionally require arthroscopic investigation and perhaps patellofemoral "shaving" if true chondromalacia is present. The vast majority of patients have an expectant benign prognosis.

Osgood–Schlatter disease

Osgood–Schlatter disease is an eponym for a condition described by these authors nearly 90 years ago. It is one of the most frequently encountered pain syndromes of adolescence, and is most commonly seen in males (roughly three to one to females). Nearly one half of the cases are bilateral. The etiology of the condition is mechanical, and it is basically a tendonitis of the distal insertion of the infrapatellar tendon. It may be accompanied by a minute avulsion fracture of the cartilaginous or bony "tongue" epiphysis of the upper tibia. The anterior portion of the upper tibial epiphysis has a "tongue-like" shape and serves as the site of insertion for the distal end of the patellar tendon. With repetitive contracture of the quadriceps mechanism a small fragment of bone or cartilage may be elevated from the distal portion of the proximal tibial epiphysis, and may secondarily induce an associated inflammatory process within the tendon, or around the tendon surface (Figure 5.16). Clinically the youngsters present

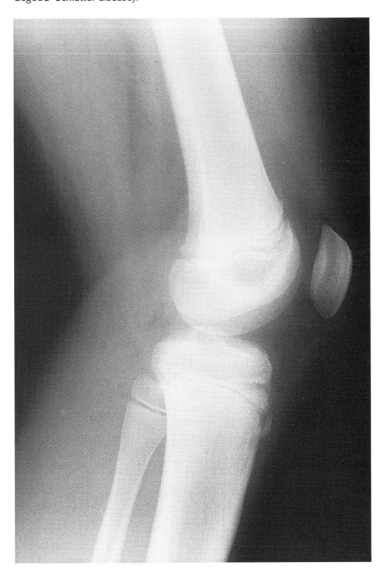

Figure 5.16. Lateral radiograph showing ossification within the upper tibial epiphysis not uncommonly seen in association with Osgood–Schlatter disease (such ossification occurs in normal children and is not diagnostic of Osgood–Schlatter disease).

with pain in the anterior aspect of the proximal tibia, characteristically aggravated by running, jumping, or knee squats. The pain is clearly mechanical in nature, and diminishes with rest. There is no evidence of intraarticular pathology on examination, and the pain is reproduced by direct compression over the bony prominence at the site of insertion of the patellar tendon (Figure 5.17).

Although radiographs are routinely obtained and may, on occasion, provide some useful information concerning other knee pathology, the diagnosis is a clinical one and should not rest with radiographs. Findings commonly associated with Osgood–Schlatter disease are bony ossicles or fragmentation of the anterior tibial epiphysis and irregularities of the ossification center.

Treatment is conservative, and routinely effective inasmuch as the disorder subsides on fusion of the upper tibial epiphysis to the shaft to the metaphysis. Once skeletal maturity is obtained it is extremely rare to encounter any cases of this condition. Ice, heat, and nonsteroidal anti-inflammatory agents combined with restriction in physical activities, particularly running, jumping, and knee squats, generally result in relief within six to eight weeks. Occasionally physiotherapy, steroid injections and casting may be necessary for recalcitrant cases. Tendon degeneration associated with the use of steroids is related to the number of injections and the amount of steroid. Casting is extremely effective, but is associated with quadriceps atrophy, and requires an almost equal time regaining strength as the time placed within the cast. Activity restrictions are generally not instituted unless the pain becomes of such a nature as to interfere with leisure time activities. For only the rarest of cases, in which a youngster has completed skeletal maturity and has radiographic demonstration of a small, ununited osseous fragment within the substance of the epiphysis with chronic recalcitrant pain, is surgical excision possibly

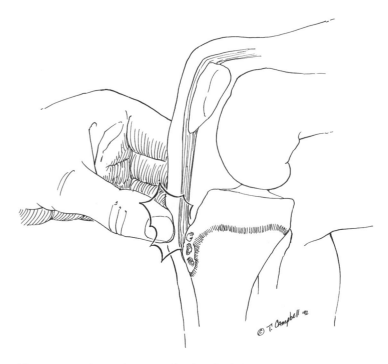

Figure 5.17. Point tenderness at the site of pain in Osgood–Schlatter disease.

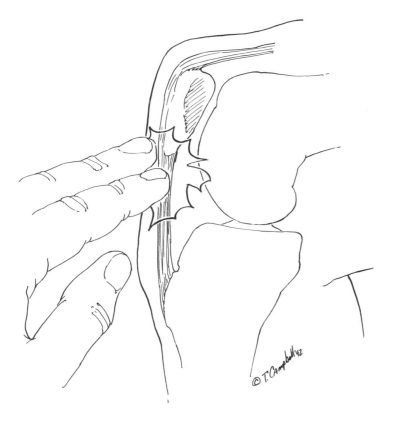

Figure 5.18. The site of point tenderness in infrapatellar tendinitis.

indicated. In its usual presentation, this clinical syndrome can be appropriately managed by primary care physicians with orthopedic referral ensuing for more chronic recalcitrant cases. The benign natural history is to be emphasized.

Infrapatellar tendinitis ("jumper's knee")

"Jumper's knee," or infrapatellar tendonitis, is a very common cause of pain during the adolescent and puberty years. It is seen in both sexes and is commonly bilateral. As with Osgood–Schlatter disease, it is a tendonitis affecting the proximal attachment of the infrapatellar tendon to the inferior pole of the patella. Secondary to chronic mechanical stress, exquisite pain, tenderness, and occasionally swelling develop in a localized area at the inferior pole of the patella (Figure 5.18). As determined by history, the pain is mechanical in nature, relieved by rest, and often relieved by the use of ice, heat, nonsteroidal anti-inflammatory medication, physical therapy, and periodic curtailment of activities, particularly running and jumping.

The natural history is for resolution to be expected by conservative methods. Well over 90 percent of all patients will obtain pain relief by non-operative means. Occasionally corticosteroid injections and casting become necessary. Activity restrictions may be implemented for those with exquisite pain and difficulty in performing routine activities, but should be reserved for only those cases. Commonly the patients will experience pain relief with the knee in extension rather than flexion. In very rare recalcitrant cases that have failed all previous conservative treatment, surgical removal of a portion of the inferior pole of the patella at the site of the tendon attachment may be necessary. Treatment is well within the domain of the primary care physician, with orthopedic referral reserved for those cases failing conservative regimens.

Calcaneal apophysitis (Sever's disease)

Calcaneal apophysitis is the most common cause of heel pain in adolescents and teenagers. It is seen equally in both sexes and is quite commonly bilateral. Although previously thought to be an osteochondritis, it is clearly a mechanical pain syndrome more closely related to a tendinitis with a self-limited benign prognosis.

As the calcaneal apophysis begins to progressively ossify at the time of adolescence, it commonly arises from more than one center of ossification and presents as a very dense radiographic pattern not unlike that seen in other osteochondritic processes (Figure 5.19). Because of this apparent fragmentation and increased density seen on the radiograph, it was thought for many years to represent a form of osteochondritis, when in fact it has been clearly shown that this is the normal pattern of ossification for this apophysis.

The youngsters in this age group will complain of pain in their heel, particularly with mechanical activities. Running and jumping generally accentuate the symptoms. The most characteristic distinguishing feature on physical examination is exquisite pain produced on medial and lateral compression of the heel at the site where the calcaneal apophysis attaches to the main body of the calcaneus (Figure 5.20). This pain is not on plantar pressure, or posterior or retrocalcaneal pressure, but on medial and lateral compression. Radiographs are generally performed to exclude other disease processes.

The natural history is for eventual symptom resolution in all cases. The symptoms resolve once the calcaneal apophysis amalgamates with the main body of the calcaneus. A simple in-shoe orthotic, consisting of a soft material covered by leather that will slightly raise the heel and cushion the impact of weight bearing, will generally result in pain relief within six weeks to three months. The elevated pad also tends to relax the gastroc-soleus complex and releases tension on the calcaneal apophysis.

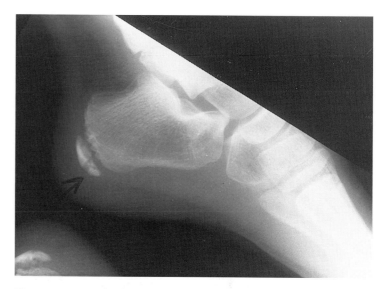

Figure 5.19. Lateral radiograph of the foot demonstrating normal irregular ossification and sclerosis within the calcaneal apophysis.

Figure 5.20. The classic site of discomfort on medial lateral compression of the heel in calcaneal apophysitis.

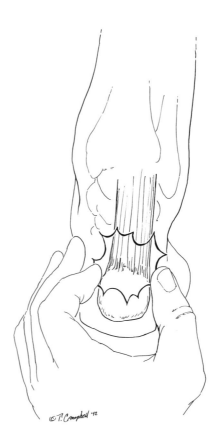

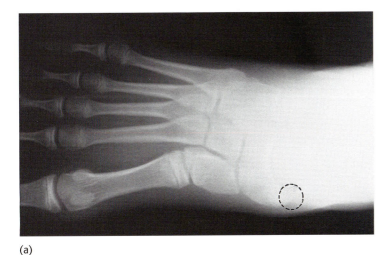

(a)

(b)

Figure 5.21. (a) Radiograph showing an accessory navicular lying proximal and medial to the navicular. (b) Lateral radiograph showing accessory navicular lying proximal to the navicular.

There is no sound reason to restrict activities and, in fact, activities are encouraged with the device. The author's personal preference is for a sponge-filled, leather-covered compressible heel pad that compresses down to five-eighths of an inch and is transferable into alternative shoe wear. In less than 10 percent of cases, a short leg plantar flexion cast, worn for three to four weeks, may be necessary. The benign natural history should be emphasized for parents. Properly recognized, this condition can often be managed by primary care physicians.

Accessory navicular (chronic posterior tibial tendinitis)

Slightly more than 10 percent of humans possess an accessory tarsal navicular. In roughly two percent of all adults the accessory navicular persists as a complete and separate ossicle unattached to the ossified navicular and embedded in the substance of the posterior tibial tendon. The etiology of the syndrome seen in adolescence and puberty is directly related to a chronic posterior tibial tendinitis occurring in association with an accessory navicular (Figures 5.21a, b). Not uncommonly a very prominent medial "cornuate-shaped" navicular may produce similar posterior tibial tendinitis in the absence of any ossified supernumerary bone.

The symptoms encountered at this age are pain with weight bearing, and difficulty in finding comfortable shoe wear. The pain is clearly mechanical in nature and generally resolves with rest. On examination, a medial prominence is encountered at the site of the proximal medial portion of the navicular, with tenderness commonly seen along the posterior tibial tendon as it reaches its insertion onto the navicular. There may be erythema and swelling as well. When pressure is applied to the plantar-medial portion of the bony prominence, exquisite pain is elicited, mimicking the patient's symptoms (Figure 5.22).

It was originally thought that the discomfort occurred because of a marked pronovalgus (flatfoot) deformity accompanying the accessory navicular. The pain was thought to arise from chronic pressure due to flattening of the longitudinal arch in the presence of a weak posterior tibial tendon. This explanation is untenable in light of the fact that the majority of patients with this condition do not have significant pronovalgus feet.

It is likely that fewer than half of the patients with this accessory ossicle have sufficient pain to seek medical attention. Treatment initially should be conservative in nature and consist of a sponge-filled long arch orthotic that can be transferred from shoe to shoe in conjunction with anti-inflammatories and physiotherapy modalities. Although cortisone injections have been utilized, they are not commonly successful, are extremely painful, and carry a small risk of infection. Occasionally below-knee casts have been temporarily successful. For patients with recalcitrant symptoms who have failed conservative care, surgical excision of the accessory navicular or the prominent medial "cornuate-shaped" navicular with plication of the posterior tibial tendon may be necessary. Surgical excision has been successful in well over 90 percent of those cases requiring surgery.

Peroneal tendinitis

Peroneal tendinitis is a fairly common cause of pain affecting the lateral border of the foot. It is most frequently seen during adolescence and occurs in both sexes equally. Bilateral cases are common. The condition is generally seen in association with a very prominent base of the fifth metatarsal. It may be difficult initially to differentiate peroneal tendinitis from an incomplete avulsion fracture of the base of the fifth metatarsal. Both conditions will present with mechanical type pain in the area of the base of the fifth metatarsal, aggravated by running and jumping. Avulsion fractures will produce a transverse radiolucent line across

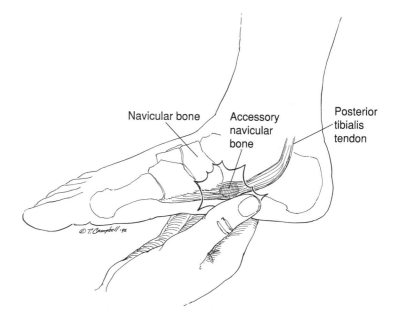

Figure 5.22. The location of point tenderness in posterior tibial tendinitis associated with an accessory navicular bone.

the base of the fifth metatarsal. Cases of peroneal tendinitis will have tenderness at the site of insertion of the tendon on the base of the fifth metatarsal, and likely along the distal tendon attachment, but radiographic changes will be absent.

The condition is self-limited with an excellent long-term prognosis. Pain relief can usually be obtained by fashioning a contoured custom-designed orthotic, transferable in nature and composed of a soft material such as sponge enveloped within a leather covering. This soft orthotic should also be fashioned so as to weight-relieve beneath the base of the fifth metatarsal during weight bearing. With an appropriately fitting orthotic, pain relief can generally be expected to occur within a six- to eight-week period. The device is effective for recurrences as well. Surgical treatment should be completely unnecessary. If there is comfort with the diagnosis, this condition certainly can be managed by primary care physicians.

Anserine bursitis

Bursae are potential spaces usually lined by synovium and designed anatomically to reduce friction during musculotendinous activity. The anserine bursa lies proximal and just medial to the midline of the upper portion of the tibia. The term anserine ("goose's foot"), relates to the peculiar anatomic configuration of the insertion of the tendons of the sartorius, gracilis, and the semitendonosis as they gain entry onto the upper medial portion of the tibia. The tendons with their investing synovial sheath lie adjacent to the bursa.

The source of pain in this region is a mechanical tendinitis arising from repetitive rotary movements of the tibia on the femur, particularly along the medial aspect of the knee. The condition is commonly seen in people involved in "twisting" motions at the knee, such as football players, runners, gymnasts, and ballet dancers. It is usually unilateral, although there are occasional cases of bilaterality. Bilateral cases should prompt investigations into inflammatory arthropathies, particularly juvenile rheumatoid arthritis. It is also seen in association with osteochondromas of the upper proximal medial tibia, but the vast majority of cases are of the pure mechanical type.

Most typically the pain is seen with mechanical activities, particularly running and twisting of the knee. Occasionally swelling and erythema may be noted. Pressure applied directly over the tendons themselves at their site of insertion will reproduce the pain (Figure 5.23). In the absence of an underlying osteochondroma, the treatment is generally conservative, and will nearly always result in resolution of symptoms. Ice, heat, in concert with nonsteroidal anti-inflammatory medication combined with occasional periods of activity restriction or physiotherapy, will generally result in pain relief within six weeks to three months. Occasionally, corticosteroid injections or casting may be necessary. Surgery must be considered meddlesome, except in cases of underlying bony pathology.

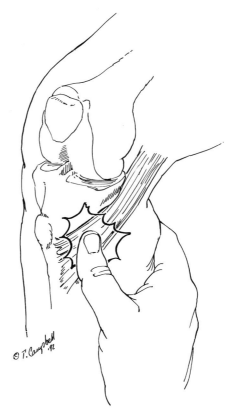

Figure 5.23. The site of point tenderness in anserine bursitis.

Fabella syndrome

In roughly 12 percent of humans, a sesamoid bone is found imbedded in the tendinous portion of the lateral head of the gastrocnemius muscle, directly adjacent and posterior to the lateral femoral condyle and commonly articulating with the condyle itself (Figures 5.24a, b and 5.25). The fabella ("little bean") has been associated with a chronic intermittent type pain in the posterolateral aspect of the knee most commonly seen in adolescence and puberty. The majority of reported cases have been in females although males are subject to the same condition. The pain is mechanical in nature, accentuated by knee extension and localized to the posterolateral portion of the popliteal fossa.

On clinical examination direct compression over the lateral head of the gastrocnemius tendon at its site of insertion onto the lateral condyle will exquisitely reproduce the

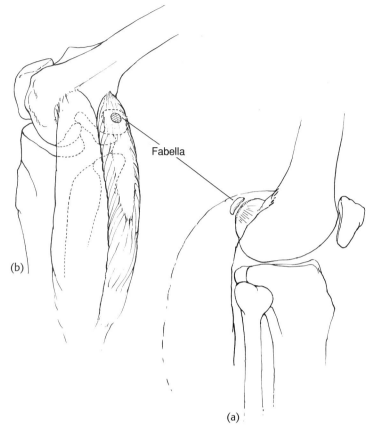

Figure 5.24. (a) The location of fabella within the lateral gastrocnemius tendon. (b) The relationship of the fabella to the lateral femoral condyle.

symptoms. The syndrome is associated with an ossified sesamoid bone in the majority of cases, although it can occur in association with a cartilaginous fragment or even in association with a thickened tendon. The source of the pain remains obscure, although it may evolve from a localized synovitis much like in the patellofemoral compression pain syndrome. Simple conservative methods combined with temporary restriction of activities and occasional corticosteroid injections have produced satisfactory results in roughly half of the cases. Recalcitrant cases with intermittent recurring pain and inability to perform leisure time activities have led to surgical removal of a portion of the lateral gastrocnemius tendon and sesamoid, if present. The results of surgery, although uncommonly required, have been successful in well over 90 percent of cases. Failure to obtain initial pain relief within a six- to eight-week period should prompt appropriate orthopedic referral.

Osteochondritis dissecans

Osteochondritis dissecans is a pain syndrome of adolescence primarily affecting the knee, secondarily the ankle, and occasionally the elbow involving the humeral capitellum. It is basically a disorder in which a segment of articular cartilage and subchondral bone becomes at least radiographically separated from the surrounding bone and cartilage. The osteochondritis dissecans fragment may remain totally in continuity with the adjacent bone and cartilage from which it arises, may be partially separated, or may become a completely loose fragment.

The etiology of osteochondritis dissecans is unknown, although several theories have been proposed. A hereditary background is noted in many cases, and it is uncommon to have more than one location within the appendicular skeleton. Trauma has been routinely implicated, and probably is etiologic in a number of cases. Localized ischemia to the area has been theorized, but has not been supported by appropriate histopathologic studies. In some cases avascular necrosis of the subchondral bone in the fragment is noted, and in others the bone is perfectly normal. Undoubtedly some cases, involving the femoral condyles, represent tertiary ossification centers, particularly in the lateral portion of the medial femoral condyle. The condition is more common in the male in roughly a three to one ratio. Without question the femoral condyle has provided the greatest number of cases.

Clinically the presenting complaints are that of pain of a mechanical nature, joint swelling, "popping," and occasional "locking" of the joint. Symptoms of "giving way" are commonly encountered. In lesions involving the lateral portion of the medial femoral condyle, rotational knee pain is commonly experienced (Figure 5.26). In lesions of the humeral capitellum, swelling of the elbow, "locking" and pain on rotation of the forearm are common (Figure 5.27). In lesions involving the dome of the talus, swelling, stiffness, locking, and particularly pain on weight bearing are most common.

Physical findings are relative to the appropriate joint. In the knee joint an effusion may be present. Pain on internal rotation of the tibia during the last 30 degrees of extension of the knee is a common finding, particularly in lesions of the lateral portion of the medial femoral condyle. With condylar fragments, direct compression over the femoral condyle with the knee fully flexed may produce pain. At the ankle and elbow levels joint effusions are common, with pain on attempts to dorsiflex, plantarflex, rotate, or invert the ankle. With lesions involving the humeral capitellum, pain is experienced with rotation of the forearm and with flexion and extension. If the osteochondritis dissecans fragment has become detached, "locking" of the joint is common.

The diagnosis is established by radiographs. Commonly a crescent-shaped radiolucent zone separates the osteochondritis fragment from the main body of the bone. Although

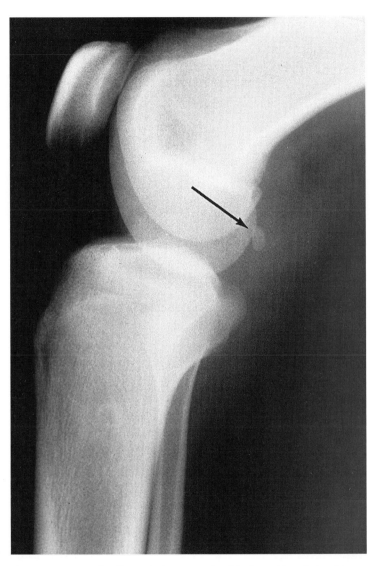

Figure 5.25. Lateral radiograph demonstrating fabella and its relationship to the lateral femoral condyle.

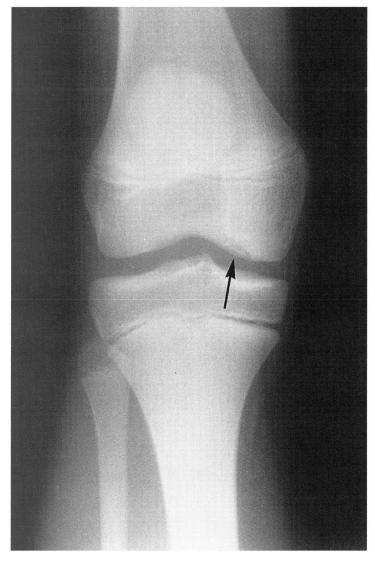

Figure 5.26. Anteroposterior radiograph demonstrating osteochondritis dissecans of the medial femoral condyle.

radiographs are the simplest and single most valuable means of identifying the osteochondritis dissecans, computed tomography is of particular significant value in localizing certain lesions (talus). Magnetic resonance imaging can provide additional information, particularly with regard to the cartilaginous surfaces and the possible presence of avascular necrosis and degree of detachment.

The natural history of the disorder is related to the location within the body and within the bone itself. At the knee level and with lesions of the lateral or medial intercondylar portion of the femoral condyles, the prognosis is generally excellent. Over 90 percent of patients with symptoms in this region will resolve their symptoms without detachment of the fragment. Condylar (weight bearing surface) lesions involving the articular portion of the femoral condyle have a somewhat worse prognosis, as would be suspected. Lesions of the humeral capitellum are often associated with recurrent episodes of pain and nearly half of these lesions eventually will require some sort of surgical procedure.

Conservative treatment should still be the mainstay. Lesions of the medial or lateral dome of the talus will occasionally resolve by conservative methods, but a high percentage of these lesions will also eventually require surgical treatment because of the constant wear and tear encountered during routine weight bearing. Many of these lesions are associated with excessive ankle ligament laxity. Surgical treatment takes the form of replacement of the fragment with stabilization, drilling and fenestration to enhance additional blood supply, and occasionally removal of a loose fragment. Orthopedic referral after recognition is recommended.

Periostitis ("shin splints")

Periostitis, or "shin splints," are symptoms commonly seen during the puberty period and rarely thereafter. A variety of other terms

currently utilized include medial tibial stress
syndrome, stress fracture, and chronic exertion
compartment syndrome. Although the
condition has never been substantiated
histopathologically or biochemically, it is
clearly a clinical entity, and of particular
importance to youngsters engaged in athletics.
It can be further characterized as doing "too
much," "too soon" and "too fast." It is generally
categorized as a form of the mechanical
overuse "stress syndromes" of the lower
extremity; the most well recognized being a
true "stress fracture." It is currently accepted as
a "stage" of progression to stress fractures. It is
seen more commonly in males but occurs in
females as well. It is nearly always associated
with significant mechanical stress in the calf,
usually related to excessive running or
jumping. The pain experienced is routinely
along the anterior medial border of the tibial
shaft directly at the site of attachment for the
anterior calf muscles as they attach onto the
periosteum of the bone. It usually begins at the
start of the activity and persists well beyond
cessation. It has been described as a sharp or
aching disabling type of pain that becomes
worse with activity and worse with ankle
dorsiflexion. Patients experience local
tenderness along the anterior medial tibial
margin at the site of muscle attachment. There
is rarely any swelling in this area and no
superficial skin changes.

The major condition to be differentiated is a
stress fracture. Radiographic evaluation, often
combined with radionuclide imaging, is of
most help. Radionuclide imaging has been
most helpful in defining stages of the stress
syndrome. "Shin splints" are often difficult to
manage and almost always necessitate
restriction of the activity that accentuated the
pain. Ice, heat, nonsteroidal anti-inflammatory
medications and physiotherapy modalities
have been helpful, but curtailment of activity
remains most important

Unfortunately, many cases occur in very
active adolescents who are psychologically
impacted by the imposed activity restrictions.

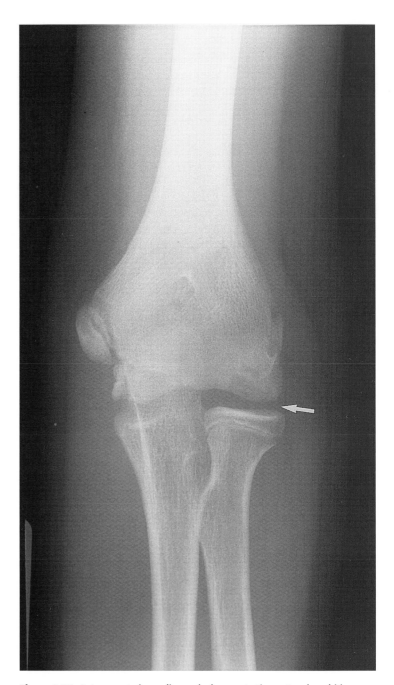

Figure 5.27. Anteroposterior radiograph demonstrating osteochondritis dissecans (Panner's disease) of the humeral capitellum.

It is also important to differentiate this entity from an exercise-induced early compartment syndrome of the anterior calf muscles, and intramuscular compartment pressures may need to be obtained. For all these reasons, orthopedic consultation is recommended in most cases.

Rotator cuff tendonitis of the shoulder

Rotator cuff tendonitis of the shoulder is generally seen during the latter part of the puberty years and much more commonly in males. It is usually unilateral, and is usually found in direct relationship to the arm undergoing the majority of athletic activity. The vast majority of youngsters seen in this age group are involved in athletic activities where throwing or hitting is the major component. Consequently baseball players, football players, track and field athletes, tennis players, and occasionally swimmers are most commonly affected. It is generally believed that repeated stress (microtrauma) in the abducted externally rotated position and the abducted internally rotated position is responsible for most of the cases. From repeated stresses on the rotator cuff an inflammatory tendonitis develops, much like the adult counterpart. Diagnosis is generally established by the presence of exquisite pain at the outer acromion on resisted abduction of the shoulder, particularly in the range from 30 degrees of abduction to 90 degrees of abduction. Radiographs to eliminate other causes of shoulder pain are indicated but are of little help in the diagnosis.

It is highly unlikely that patients in the second decade would have actual tearing of the rotator cuff so commonly seen in older patients, although histologic documentation is unavailable. Whether or not repeated episodes of rotator cuff tendinitis in the adolescent years leads to long-term rotator cuff tears is controversial. Magnetic resonance imaging may be helpful to differentiate actual tears.

The natural history in adolescents and teenagers is much more benign than in the adult, with the majority of cases responding to conservative care consisting of ice, heat, nonsteroidal anti-inflammatory medications, physiotherapy modalities and periods of rest. Activities can be readily resumed once the inflammatory reaction subsides and strength returns. Pain relief is generally obtained in three to six weeks with rapid return of strength to be expected. Failures of initial management may necessitate orthopedic referral.

Epicondylitis ("tennis elbow")

"Tennis elbow" is seen occasionally in late teenagers, particularly in athletes, more commonly in males, and more commonly in baseball pitchers and tennis players. It may occur at either the medial or lateral epicondyle or even occasionally at the triceps insertion onto the olecranon. Regardless of its location the treatment is identical. The condition occurs as a result of repetitive minute (overuse) stresses delivered at the tendinous insertion onto the bone, thereby producing a localized tendinitis and inflammatory reaction. It is easily diagnosable by palpation and reproduction of the patient's symptoms (Figure 5.28). Occasionally a radiohumeral bursitis may mimic a lateral epicondylitis (both forms of tennis elbow), but the distinction is of academic interest only. Ice, heat, nonsteroidal anti-inflammatory medications, physiotherapy modalities, periods of relief from stress and the use of a forearm orthotic generally will result in a satisfactory result within six weeks to three months. Occasionally injections of corticosteroids may be necessary. Surgery is almost always reserved for patients beyond the second decade with recalcitrant symptoms.

Iliotibial band syndrome ("snapping hip")

Iliotibial band tendinitis or "snapping hip" is seen in the teenage–late adolescent. It is almost exclusively found in females, and is a result of a tendinitis directly related to impingement of the iliotibial band across the greater

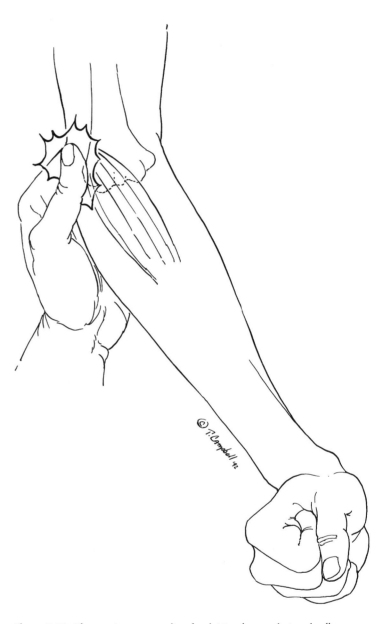

Figure 5.28. The most common site of point tenderness in tennis elbow.

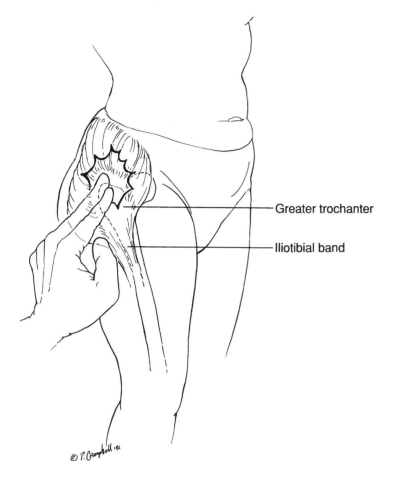

Figure 5.29. Point tenderness over greater trochanter at the site of "snapping hip."

trochanteric ridge. As the pelvis in females expands and widens at the time of puberty, the greater trochanter becomes quite prominent in many females. The iliotibial band will become tautly draped across the greater trochanter and from repetitive flexion-extension and rotation movements of the hip a tendinitis develops at the site where the tendon lies directly adjacent to the greater trochanter. The iliotibial band may thicken and may actually produce a "snapping" or "popping" sensation as the tendon migrates back and forth across the trochanteric ridge. The "snapping" may be even sufficiently audible to frighten the patient into believing the hip is actually dislocating. Diagnosis is readily established by the direct reproduction of symptoms by palpation and compression over the trochanter during hip joint motions (Figure 5.29). The patient may be voluntarily able to produce the "snapping."

Once the diagnosis is established treatment is conservative, and in well over 95 percent of all cases is successful. Treatment consists of ice, heat, nonsteroidal anti-inflammatory medications, physiotherapy modalities and periods of restriction of physical activities, particularly those directly related to symptom augmentation. Occasionally injections of corticosteroids have been helpful. In less than one percent of all cases surgery has been found necessary, and consists of division of the fibers of the iliotibial band that come in direct contact with the greater trochanter.

Freiberg's infraction

Freiberg's infraction, described over 80 years ago, consists of an osteochondritis of the head of the second metatarsal and occasionally the third metatarsal. Histopathologically it has been identified as an avascular necrosis of the metatarsal head. The condition presents as a painful metatarsalgia localized over the involved metatarsal head. Swelling is usually present and the pain is exacerbated by weight bearing and particularly by running and jumping. It is seen at the time of puberty and is more common in the female, with well over three-quarters of all cases occurring in females. The actual etiology is unknown, but it may be related to the peculiar anatomic exposure to stress concentration on the second metatarsal head during repetitive weight bearing stresses in certain foot configurations. It is likely that trauma plays a significant role. The diagnosis is established by standard radiographs, occasionally combined with radionuclide imaging (Figure 5.30).

The natural history is for eventual pain relief to occur in the vast majority of cases regardless of treatment. Treatment is generally indicated because of the significant pain with weight bearing, and consists of brief periods of immobilization in a short leg cast, followed by weight relief from an in-shoe soft orthotic designed to shift weight bearing off the appropriate metatarsal head. Less than 10 percent of the cases become recalcitrant to conservative methods and require surgical treatment. Once the diagnosis is established it is generally acceptable for orthopedic referral to ensue shortly thereafter.

"Ingrown" toenails

"Ingrown" toenails are a very common cause of pain in the foot in adolescents and teenagers. They are seen equally in both sexes and arise from a consistent etiology. The lateral and distal margins of the medial and lateral portion of the great toenail are allowed to invaginate beneath the skin margins. The paronychial skin then grows over the nail both distally and proximally and incarcerates the nail below and within (Figure 5.31). Bacteria and debris accumulate beneath the paronychial margins and infection develops, supplemented by repeated trauma from the overlying pressure from the sock and shoe. The paronychial infection blossoms, spreads, and produces erythema, increased edema and exquisite pain. Diagnosis is rarely in doubt, and radiographs should be obtained only to make sure that

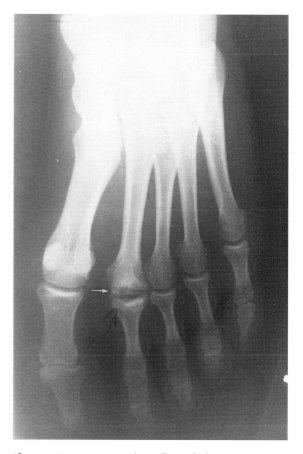

Figure 5.30. Anteroposterior radiograph demonstrating Freiberg's infraction of the second metatarsal head.

Figure 5.31. Ingrown great toenail with paronychial hypertrophy and infection.

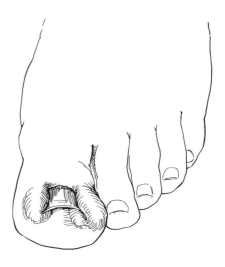

there is no phalangeal osteomyelitis. Initial treatment consists of warm soaks, local debridement usually with a cotton swab and an antiseptic solution, combined with loose fitting foot coverings, in concert with appropriate antibiotics when necessary. Failure to resolve is common and surgical treatment is often necessary. A number of surgical techniques are available and appropriate orthopedic referral should be obtained.

"Pump bumps"

"Pump bumps" are the lay term for what is essentially a reactive calcaneal osteocartilaginous prominence. They are bony prominences protruding directly from the posterior–superior portion of the apophysis of the os calcis occurring under and directly adjacent to the Achilles tendon insertion. The term arose from the pain syndrome associated with the wear of high countered women's fashion shoes (pumps) seen in years past. The constant "rubbing" from the counter produced a reactive change in the calcaneal apophysis resulting in what appeared to be an osteocartilaginous "lump." The bony prominences occur either on one side of the Achilles tendon or both and can produce exquisite tenderness (Figure 5.32). Radiographs fail to reveal any true bony lesion other than a bony prominence in the painful region. Localized erythema and edema (bursitis) usually accompany the localized tenderness.

The natural history is benign in most cases, symptoms are often ameliorated by simply altering shoe wear. Occasionally soft in-shoe orthotics beneath the heel may shift the painful area away from the counter of the shoe. In less than 10 percent of cases that have been resistant to treatment, surgery may be necessary, consisting of resection of the bony prominence. Inasmuch as the results of surgery have not infrequently been disappointing, it is to be viewed as a last resort as the painful lump may be replaced by a painful scar.

Figure 5.32. The osteocartilaginous prominence seen in association with "pump bumps" and the presumed etiology.

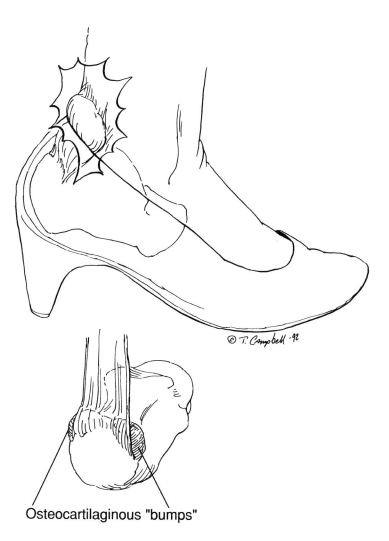

© T. Campbell '92

Osteocartilaginous "bumps"

de Quervain's disease

de Quervain's disease is an inflammatory tendinitis of the wrist affecting the extensor pollicis brevis and the abductor pollicis. The origins of the painful symptoms appear to be a by-product of an inflammatory process within the tendon sheath at the site where the tendons cross the wrist. The tendons run in a grooved bony tunnel that is often fairly narrow in dimension. Repetitive irritations of the tendons in this localized region may result in inflammation with swelling of the tendons and the peritendinous tissues, thereby providing little room within the tunnel for movement. Pain in the wrist and weakness of the hand and wrist are common presenting symptoms. The condition appears at the time of puberty and is slightly more common in females. People engaged in repetitive wrist motion have a greater susceptibility (clerical workers, surgeons, writers).

Diagnosis is readily established by direct compression at the distal end of the radius combined with a positive Finkelstein test. The Finkelstein test consists of a forced volar flexion and ulnar deviation of the thumb at both metacarpophalangeal and interphalangeal joints and at wrist level. Reproduction of exquisite pain is elicited at the site on the distal radius of the narrow tunnel (Figure 5.33).

Treatment consists of temporary immobilization combined with ice, heat, and nonsteroidal anti-inflammatory medications. Treatment is generally successful in adolescents and teenagers within a six-week to three-month time period. Failures may require corticosteroid injection and occasionally surgical division of the enveloping constricting fibrous sheath. Surgery is indicated in a small number of cases and is not always successful. Appropriate diagnosis should be followed by orthopedic referral in most cases.

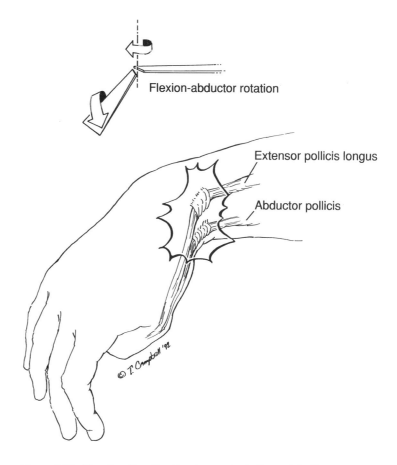

Flexion-abductor rotation

Extensor pollicis longus

Abductor pollicis

© T. Campbell '92

Figure 5.33. The site of localized tenderness in de Quervain's disease (Finkelstein test).

Chapter 6

Miscellaneous disorders

It is that which we do know which is the greatest
hindrance to our learning that which we do not know.
Bernard

The limping child

This section has been included to provide a
useful, brief characterization of the sources of
limp in childhood and adolescence. Although
not designed to be fully comprehensive, it
hopefully will provide a simple checklist for the
physician. The causes of limp will be discussed
in three age groups: age one to three years;
three to ten years; and adolescence and
puberty.

There are two basic types of limps seen in
children: weakness limp and antalgic (painful)
limp. A third type of limp is seen in concert with
leg length discrepancy and is actually a tilting
of one side of the pelvis, as an accommodation
of the short leg to the long leg, rather than a
true limp. A limp resulting from muscle
weakness is characterized by a prolonged
stance phase of gait, or in other words, a longer
period of time during single limb support to
allow the body to compensate for the muscle
weakness. An antalgic limp is characterized by
a very short stance phase, further defined by a
reluctance of the individual to stay on the part
that hurts any longer than is necessary. In
general, antalgic or painful limps come from
the hip, knee, or foot and ankle, and their
attached parts. It is often an academic detective
game to discern the exact source of the limp.

In an antalgic limp arising from the hip, the patient plants the affected limb on the ground, and leans laterally over the hip, thereby centralizing the body's center of gravity directly over the femoral head and shaft of the femur and distributing the weight in a more diffuse fashion along the entire limb (Figure 6.1). Characteristically, the youngster rapidly leans over the hip and gets off the limb rapidly. In an antalgic limp arising from the knee, the knee is characteristically bent, the body leans away from the affected limb, the foot is planted on the ground quickly, and weight bearing occurs instantly on and off, shifting the trunk weight onto the normal limb (Figure 6.2). In an antalgic limp arising from pathology within the foot and ankle, the patient leans the body toward the opposite normal extremity, touches the foot and ankle down just briefly, and weight shifts immediately onto the opposite side (Figure 6.3). It is important to remember that in the painful type of limp there is a very short stance phase, in contrast with a muscle weakness type of limp in which there is a very prolonged stance phase, and a lengthy period of single limb weight support.

The history relative to the limp is quite important, as limping may have diurnal variations, may be persistent or intermittent in nature, may have been in close association with a recent illness, may have a peculiar type of appearance, and may be significantly affected by ascending and descending stairs. It is useful to do a very thorough clinical evaluation, particularly with "laying on of hands." Palpation of the affected part will commonly reveal the source. Standing on one leg or both legs, walking fore and aft, and attempts at running will all be useful. Placing joints through a range of motion is essential in evaluating subtle degrees of stiffness and joint effusion. Adjunctive studies are of the essence, and include appropriate laboratory tests, conventional radiography, and radionuclide imaging. A quick review of a pathology "checklist" will help orient the various conditions seen in the various age groups, and

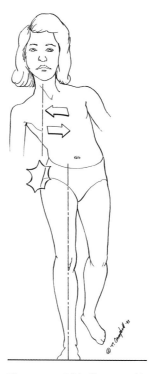

Figure 6.1. A hip limp at midstance. Trunk shifts over the hip quickly, and then shifts back to the opposite side.

Figure 6.2. A painful knee limp with the trunk shifting away from the involved extremity at midstance.

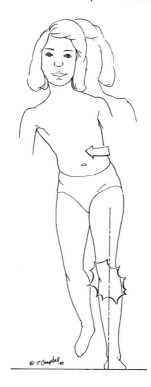

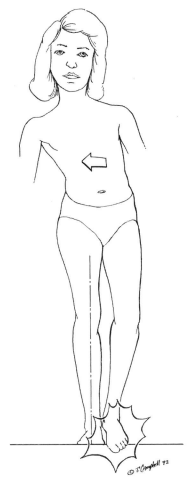

Figure 6.3. A painful foot limp with trunk shifting away from the involved extremity at midstance.

will incorporate the categories of trauma, infection, inflammation, circulatory disorders, congenital disorders, paralytic disorders, metabolic disorders and neoplastic disorders. Without question in all of the age groups encountered in children and adolescents, trauma is the number one etiologic factor. One of the more common causes of pain in children is *juvenile myalgia* or "growing pains." Long attributed to be a myth perpetuated by grandparents, it is indeed a real condition.

Between the ages of one and three years, the most common cause of a painful limp in a child is trauma, most notably fractures of the base of the first metatarsal, and of the necks of the second through the fifth metatarsals. Fractures of the tibia of the "toddler type" are seen in this age group and are usually a spiral fracture of the shaft, or a compression fracture of the distal tibia. Limping secondary to abuse must always be a part of the differential diagnosis, particularly in this age group. Conditions such as toxic synovitis of the hip or knee, and juvenile rheumatoid arthritis are seen, but are far less common. Osteomyelitis and septic arthritis are occasionally encountered. Limping from a neuromuscular origin occurs not uncommonly in this age group, particularly in the form of spastic hemiplegia.

Between the ages of 3–10 years, trauma is still the most common cause for limp. Antalgic limps of hip origin are most often seen with "toxic" or "transient" synovitis of the hip and Legg–Calvé–Perthes disease, which is far less common than "toxic" synovitis of the hip. Juvenile rheumatoid arthritis is seen in this age group, as well as osteomyelitis and occasionally septic arthritis. Between the ages of 10 years and skeletal maturity, trauma is still the number one etiology for antalgic limps. In this age group the pain syndromes of adolescence, which are adequately addressed elsewhere in the text, occupy a large proportion of the causes of limp. Slipped capital femoral epiphysis should always be primarily considered in an antalgic limp in this age group. Although other conditions are somewhat uncommon, back pain may radiate into the lower extremities with accompanying limp (Pearls 6.1, 6.2, 6.3, 6.4). A very careful history and physical examination, including direct palpation of the affected limb, will usually disclose the diagnosis in at least 90 percent of all cases of limp. Adjunctive studies such as radiography, laboratory studies, radionuclide imaging, computed tomography (CT), and magnetic resonance imaging (MRI) will generally provide the answer in more complex cases.

Leg length discrepancy

The assessment and management of leg length discrepancy has been improved by tremendous recent advances in technology relative to evaluation and treatment. Computed tomography, MRI imaging, and the enormous capacity of modern external fixation devices to achieve limb lengthening have made a previously simplistic problem into a much more complex issue but with a favorable overall impact.

The simplest technique of evaluating disparity in lower limb length is obtained by placing the index fingers on the uppermost portion of the iliac crest with the patient standing symmetrically, heels to the floor, knees in full extension, and hips in full extension. Any significant discrepancy of clinical importance can be readily detected and measured by placing blocks of wood beneath the shorter limb and balancing the pelvis (Figure 6.4). Anisomelia (unequal leg lengths) of upwards of 8–9 mm is common in well over three-quarters of all individuals. The method of measuring differences in limb length can be significantly affected by a restricted range of motion in any of the joints of the lower extremity and particularly adduction, abduction, or flexion deformity of the hip.

An additional method of limb length determination is performed by placing a measuring device (tape measure) at the anterior superior iliac spine and measuring the

Pearl 6.1. Differential diagnosis of limp (pathologic categories)

Trauma
Infection
Inflammation
Circulatory
Congenital
Paralytic
Metabolic
Neoplasia

Pearl 6.2. Most common causes of limp at age 1–3 years

Trauma
Inflammation
Infection
Paralytic

Pearl 6.3. Most common causes of limp at age 3–10 years

Trauma
"Toxic" synovitis
Legg–Calvé–Perthes
Juvenile arthritis

Pearl 6.4. Most common causes of limp at age 10 years to skeletal maturity

Trauma
Pain syndromes of adolescence
Slipped epiphysis

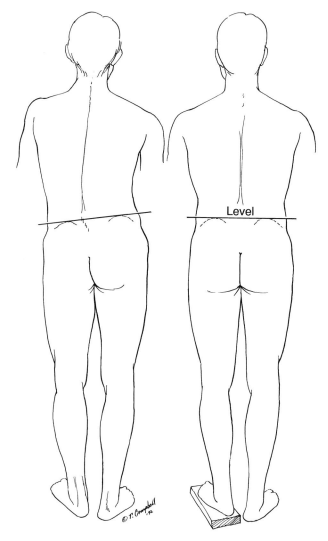

Figure 6.4. The use of blocks of wood to balance leg length inequality.

length down to the medial most distal extremity of the medial malleolus (Figure 6.5). An appropriate site at the maximum prominence of the medial femoral condyle may also be used to help determine the relative differential length between both femurs and both tibiae. Commonly, radiographic scanograms are taken of the lower extremities, which are quite helpful in differentiating relative disproportion between both femurs and both tibiae, but fail to include the pelvis and remaining ankle and foot below the lower end of the tibia.

There are numerous disorders and diseases that may cause a lower limb length inequality. Most fall under the general categories of developmental malformations, tumors or tumor-like conditions, infections of bone and joints, trauma, neuromuscular disorders, and miscellaneous acquired conditions. They are often segregated into two basic categories: those that tend to diminish longitudinal growth, and those that tend to stimulate longitudinal growth (Pearls 6.5, 6.6). Conditions that increase blood flow to growth plates will generally accelerate longitudinal bone growth and those that diminish blood flow to growth plates will decelerate longitudinal growth.

The most rapid period of growth is during the first year of life, followed by the next most rapid period of growth at the time of the adolescent growth spurt. In general, girls have accelerated bone ages roughly 18–24 months relative to boys. Accordingly the adolescent female growth spurt generally, on the average, takes place 18–24 months earlier than for males. Although there is a reasonable variance among authors concerning the time of radiographic completion of growth in males and females, in general, females have completed their skeletal maturation, on the average, by 15–15.5 years as compared with males at 16.5–17 years. Radiographic determination of skeletal maturation is believed to be accurate at a level of plus or minus six months in children 10 years or older. Bone age determination is usually based on hand radiographs compared to known standards for males and females.

Pearl 6.5. Examples of orthopedic conditions causing accelerated growth

Hemangioma
Lymphangioma
Neurofibromata
Infection
Inflammation
Trauma
Hemihypertrophy
(Wilms tumor <6 years old)

Although there are other techniques available to determine and predict the expected growth in a given portion of an extremity during puberty, a very simple technique that has been used at our institution for many years consists of determining radiographically the skeletal age of the individual, and predicting growth from the distal femoral epiphysis at 1 cm per year after the age of 10 years, and 7 mm from the proximal tibial epiphysis. Any technique used to predict expected growth within the femur and tibia in adolescence and puberty is hampered by the fact that we are unable at this point in time to determine exactly when skeletal maturation will occur. Males and females at the time of puberty may rapidly progress to early skeletal maturation or may very slowly progress to maturation, beyond average ages of expectation. This may result in errors of significance in prediction, particularly when considering surgical arrest of growth by epiphyseodesis.

There are basically four ways to approach managing leg length discrepancy (Pearl 6.7). In the vast majority of cases, limb inequality is so slight as to not even require the use of balancing devices such as shoe lifts. Most adults 162 cm in height or above can readily handle a 2 cm inequality without requiring balancing. Fortunately the vast majority of limb length inequalities fall within that level. For discrepancies under 3 cm, shoe lifts will be satisfactory for most patients. For those discrepancies 3–5 cm on the average and in those children with sufficient remaining growth prior to skeletal maturation, epiphyseodesis or surgical arrest of the appropriate growth area may be indicated. Of the surgical options available, epiphyseodesis is by far the simplest and safest. Discrepancies above that degree (6 cm plus) are generally managed by surgical lengthenings or shortenings. Lengthenings and shortenings are much more complex than epiphyseodesis, with a higher degree of associated complications. In spite of the many known complications, modern lengthening devices and techniques

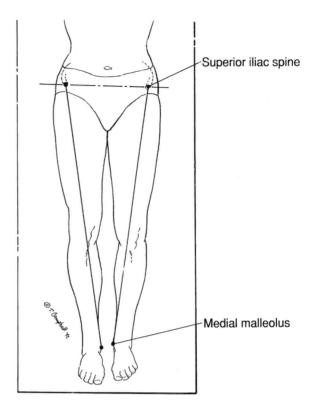

Figure 6.5. The technique of measurement from anterosuperior iliac spine to the medial malleolus.

Pearl 6.6. Examples of orthopedic conditions causing decelerated growth

Cerebral palsy
Myelodysplasia
Growth plate injury (infection)
   (Legg–Calvé–Perthes) (trauma)
Congenital hypoplasia

Pearl 6.7. Management of limb length discrepancy

<2 cm – No treatment of shoe lift
2–5 cm – Epiphyseodesis or shoe lift
6 cm ⊕ – Limb lengthening or shortening

have allowed remarkable degrees of lengthening to be achieved. The role of the primary care physician is to be aware of the means of evaluation and determination of the degree of discrepancy and the etiology of that discrepancy if possible. Clearly, the orthopedic surgeon is an obvious ally in the overall approach to management.

Arthrogryposis multiplex congenita

Arthrogryposis multiplex congenita is a non-progressive syndrome present at birth and characterized by multiple joint contractures, as a result of fibrosis of the affected soft tissues and muscles in the extremities. Although very rare, it can be devastating for function. The exact etiology is unclear and is likely multifactorial. An underlying neurologic disorder, as yet undetermined, is currently considered as the likely basic pathomechanism.

The condition is generally seen in one of three different forms. The initial type demonstrates generalized joint contractures involving primarily the limbs; a second type shows limb contractures in association with other areas of affectation of the viscera, or face and skull; and a third group has been differentiated as having congenital contractures associated with central nervous system disturbance. In the initial group of congenital joint contractures primarily involving the limbs, children are symmetrically affected with a combination of flexion and extension contractures in all limbs. There is marked apparent atrophy of muscle tissue (amyoplasia) and a tremendous reduction in active and passive motion of joints. Characteristically there are usually a few degrees of passive motion beyond the voluntarily producible range of motion. Skin creases tend to be absent and "dimpling" may be present at the joint levels. Commonly in the upper extremities, the shoulders are internally rotated, the elbows may either be flexed or extended, and the forearms are pronated with the wrists usually in flexion and the thumbs flexed into the palm (Figure 6.6a). In the lower extremities the feet are characteristically in equinovarus (clubfoot) with the knees presenting with either flexion or extension contractures and even knee dislocation. The hips may be located and lying in flexion and external rotation, or they may be dislocated (Figure 6.6b). Scoliosis, occasionally very severe, is quite common. It is important to remember that intelligence is generally normal, and treatment is designed to deal with the very severe contractures and deformities. A distal form of this basic type of involvement has been recognized, primarily involving the hands and feet, with a characteristic posturing as seen in the more extensive type.

The second type of multiple congenital joint contractures with areas of involvement of the viscera and craniofacies appears to be related to many of the "named syndromes" with similar types of extremity deformities. A much larger group of patients have multiple congenital contractures associated with central nervous system dysfunction and are commonly associated with chromosomal abnormalities. There is a very high attrition rate during the first few years of life – nearing 50 percent. Two types of presentation of this are generally recognized: a neuropathic form and a myopathic form. The neuropathic form is not only more common but is more severe. Chromosomal studies and muscle biopsies are used for differentiation. The neuropathic form is generally associated with a disorder of the anterior horn cells of the central nervous system. The myopathic form is not associated with changes in the brain or the anterior horn cells and appears to be a direct affectation of the muscle tissue with replacement thereof with fibrous and fatty tissue. The deformities seen are common to all types of arthrogryposis, and pose perplexing problems in orthopedic management.

The severe rigidity of the tissues necessitates extensive surgical releases and bony reconstructive procedures to restore

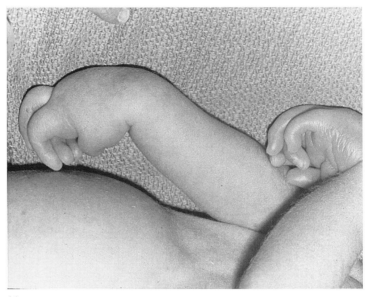

(a)

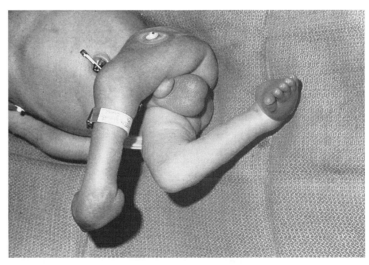

(b)

Figure 6.6. (a) Arthrogryposis multiplex congenita of the upper extremities. (b) Arthrogryposis multiplex congenita of the lower extremities.

alignment, and position the lower extremities for weight bearing. Surgery is most often directed at the lower extremities, the hand, and the management of spinal deformity. Appropriate orthopedic referral should be made following diagnosis.

Cerebral palsy

In spite of the fact that entire texts have been written about this condition, it is appropriate to include a discussion of management, particularly as it pertains to the perspectives of the pediatric orthopedist and the primary care physician. Cerebral palsy is generally defined as a non-progressive, non-transient disorder affecting the brain or spinal cord and occurring during the antenatal or early postnatal period. It is suggested that the lesion affects the developing central nervous system in a one-time fashion. Associated with the noted impairment are the obvious involvement of mentation, speech, hearing, vision, and sensation. The result of the neurologic impairment is a disturbance of movement with skeletal deformation.

Affected patients are generally classified as to the type of neurologic involvement, and as to the pattern of involvement within the trunk and extremities (Pearls 6.8, 6.9). Patients are classified as to spasticity (85–90 percent), athetosis, rigidity, tremor, and ataxia. They are also classified as to the area of involvement such as hemiplegia, diplegia (all four extremities, lowers involved more than uppers), double hemiplegia (all four extremities, one side and upper extremities more than lowers), and paraplegia. Cases of true monoplegia are occasionally seen.

In general, children affected with spasticity are more commonly aided by orthopedic measures than all other types. Hemiplegics constitute well over half of all geographic patterns of involvement, and the vast majority will eventually walk and run. Paraplegia is extremely rare, and is commonly hereditary

---

Pearl 6.8. Cerebral palsy classification by type

Spasticity (85–90%)
Athetosis
Rigidity
Tremor
Ataxia

Pearl 6.9. Cerebral palsy classification by location

Hemiplegia (>50%)
Diplegia
Double hemiplegia
Paraplegia
Monoplegia (rare)

when seen. Diplegics and double hemiplegics, when primarily spastic, also are commonly aided by orthopedic measures. The degree of mental retardation and the ability to communicate often will determine the prognosis, regardless of the type of patient.

Physicians are usually quite familiar with the establishment of the clinical diagnosis of cerebral palsy. The vast majority of cases are diagnosed between 12 and 18 months of age when a sufficient time has elapsed for the evaluation of developmental milestones. In general, hemiplegics will walk by 18–24 months of age, whereas diplegics will not walk until two to four years of age. Children with cerebral palsy achieve their normal developmental milestones later but in the same sequential pattern as normal children.

The role of the pediatric orthopedic surgeon is related to the presence and degree of disorders of motion and positioning. Commonly, affected children will have joint contractures and deformities, abnormal bone angulation and rotation, joint subluxations or dislocations, and spinal deformity. The exact indications for orthotics and the implementation of surgical treatment go beyond the scope of this book, but a few basic comments are appropriate. Hemiplegics generally are afflicted by equinus of the hindfoot and occasionally equinovarus or equinovalgus. A shortened extremity will be present on the hemiplegic side. Orthotics and/or surgical intervention may be necessary. Most recently botulinum toxin and tone reducing medications have been found effective in reducing tone in spasticity and can be helpful in delaying surgical treatment. The effects are not permanent and the overall average time of effectiveness of botulinum toxin is roughly eighteen months. Diplegics are more severely involved and usually have hindfoot equinovarus or equinovalgus, knee flexion deformity or contracture, hip flexion, adduction and internal rotation deformity, and occasionally hip subluxation and dislocation. In the hemiplegic, the upper extremity commonly will have pronation and flexion at the wrist, digital flexion, and "thumb-in-palm" flexion deformity. This is also seen in the diplegic. It is important that the pediatric orthopedic surgeon be an integral part of the overall team management of patients with cerebral palsy, particularly of the spastic type. It is recommended that appropriate orthopedic referral is obtained once the diagnosis is firmly established, particularly in spastic cerebral palsy.

Myelomeningocele (myelodysplasia)

Myelomeningocele is characterized by a failure of fusion between the developing vertebral body arches with subsequent dysplasia of the spinal cord and membranes. Experimentally, myelomeningocele can be produced by preventing closure of the neural tube, or by causing a rupture of the tube once it has already closed. The etiology is multifactorial with a hereditary background. There is a substantial incidence of appearance of the defect in subsequent offspring. Two recent advances, namely prenatal ultrasound to define the fetal spine and serum analysis to determine the presence of levels of alphafetoprotein, have facilitated antenatal diagnosis. Currently folic acid supplemental treatment is recommended in women of child-bearing age and early in pregnancy and has dramatically helped in reducing the incidence. As with cerebral palsy, the multisystem involvement of a child with myelomeningocele necessitates a medical and allied health team to optimize habilitation. The neural defect results in muscle paresis and paralysis, and the muscle imbalance leads to bone and joint deformity. Many youngsters will require surgical intervention at the soft tissue and bony level to facilitate standing or walking.

Orthopedic involvement should be obtained early to assist in the management of deformities relative to neuromuscular imbalance. The goal of orthopedic intervention is to increase independence. Scoliosis of significant magnitude is commonly seen. Higher neurologic levels (T12, L1) usually render the patient wheelchair bound, where skin problems (decubitus), osteopenia, and scoliosis dominate. The most important prognostic factor related to the ability to walk is the neurologic level. In lower levels, compatible with some form of ambulation (independent or assisted ambulation), soft tissue contractures, and osseous deformity may require surgical attention. Hip dislocation has not been definitively shown to be a significant deterrent to ambulation, particularly if bilateral. Orthotics are utilized in most patients, with patients functioning at the lower lumbar and upper sacral levels requiring the simplest and least bracing. The presence of knee extension usually implies that only short leg bracing, at the most, will be necessary. As a consequence of osteopenia (neurologic and disuse), fractures are common and decubitus ulcers can occur secondary to insensate tissue. Loss of continued ambulation in later years seems directly linked to excessive body weight.

Inasmuch as nearly all myelomeningocele patients will require periodic orthopedic, neurosurgical and urologic care as they grow, early referral is suggested from the primary care standpoint. Optimally the primary care physician should be the central coordinator of the health care team.

Sprengel's deformity

Congenital elevation of the scapula, or Sprengel's deformity, is a condition in which the scapula rests at a level much higher in the superior posterior thorax than normal. Its elevated position is believed to be the result of an error in development. The scapula, after forming in the fifth post-conception week, gradually descends from its original location opposite the fifth cervical vertebra to its adult position. In Sprengel's deformity, the scapula is small, is abnormally high in location and malrotated, and has a distorted overall shape

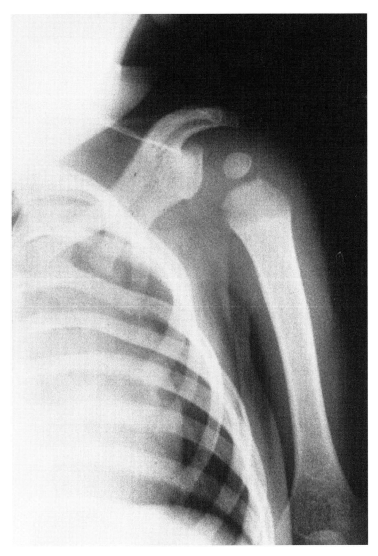

Figure 6.7. Anteroposterior radiograph showing hypoplastic scapula with superior migration.

(Figure 6.7). The superior medial angle is very prominent and is tilted anteriorly. Not uncommonly, a bony bridge (omovertebral bone) may actually attach the vertebral border of the scapula to the spinous process of the lower cervical vertebrae. The attachment of the scapula to the vertebrae may be by bone, cartilage, or by a fibrous band. The resultant high position is associated with abnormalities in all of the musculature that attaches the scapula to the thoracic wall. The clavicle is often hypoplastic. It is likewise common to see cervical ribs, cervical vertebral fusion, rib fusion, hemivertebrae, congenital scoliosis, and renal abnormalities.

Females are involved three times more often than males, and bilaterality has been reported in 10–30 percent of cases. Because of the unusual location, abduction and forward flexion of the shoulder are routinely limited as well as other rotational movements of the scapula on the thorax. Often the clinical appearance may resemble "winging" but this is due to the malrotation of the scapula in relation to the chest wall. The functional disability is related to the loss of shoulder motion, particularly abduction, and to the cosmetic deformity.

A sizable number of operations have been developed to re-establish the normal anatomic position of the scapula and its adjacent muscle, with varying degrees of success. The best surgical results have been obtained in children between three and eight years of age. Cosmetic improvement can be obtained in select cases by surgical excision of the prominence of the superomedial angle of the scapula even into adolescence and puberty. The primary care physician's role rests with establishing the diagnosis and in further defining any associated conditions.

Klippel–Feil syndrome

Klippel–Feil syndrome is essentially a fusion of two or more vertebrae in the cervical region. In its classic form it is characterized by a shortening of the neck (brevicollis) with limitation of cervical motion. The posterior hairline is generally much lower as a result of the congenital fusion (Figure 6.8). Etiologically it is a failure of normal segmentation in the cervical spine. The condition is commonly associated with a *pterygium colli* or webbing of the soft tissues on either side of the neck. Torticollis is quite common and Sprengel's deformity is seen on occasion. Much like Sprengel's deformity, it is often associated with cervical ribs, scoliosis (roughly 60 percent), congenital rib fusion, syndactyly, hypoplastic thumbs, and hypoplasia of the pectoralis major (Poland's syndrome) (Pearl 6.10). Abnormalities of the cardiovascular system, particularly septal defects, can occur and there is a very high incidence of urinary tract abnormalities. Routine investigations of the urinary tract are recommended. The diagnosis is readily established by compiling the clinical manifestations and coupling them with the radiographic appearance. The role of the primary care physician is to establish the diagnosis and define the extent of multisystem involvement. Early referral is recommended to facilitate evaluation of the spinal deformity.

Congenital dislocation of the radial head

Congenital dislocation of the radial head is a very uncommon condition in which the radial head is dislocated, usually posteriorly or laterally, and only occasionally anteriorly. It is usually unilateral but bilateral cases have been reported. It is rarely detected in early life, being recognized much later in childhood, probably as a result of the exceptionally good function usually accompanying the condition. It is often detected innocuously, either by the patient who feels a bony prominence, or by the doctor during a routine examination for other problems. The ulna is usually bowed in a direction commensurate with the direction of dislocation. Although some degree of

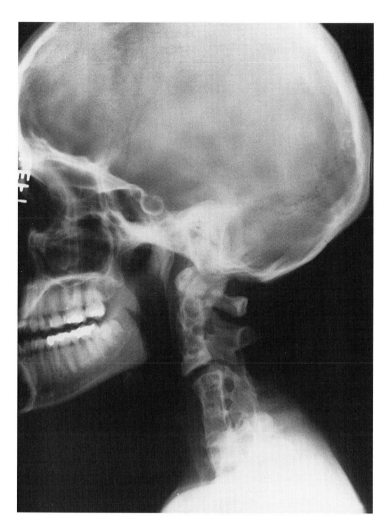

Figure 6.8. Lateral radiograph of Klippel–Feil syndrome showing multiple congenital cervical fusions.

Pearl 6.10. Associated conditions with Sprengel's deformity and Klippel–Feil syndrome

Rib and vertebral anomalies
Hand anomalies
Cardiac abnormalities
Renal abnormalities
Scoliosis

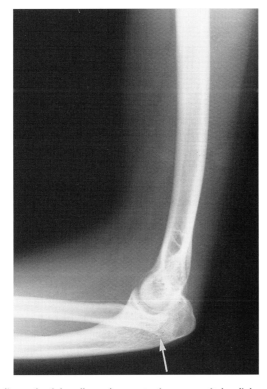

Figure 6.9. Lateral radiograph of the elbow demonstrating congenital radial head dislocation.

Figure 6.10. Lateral radiograph of the elbow illustrating proximal congenital radioulnar synostosis.

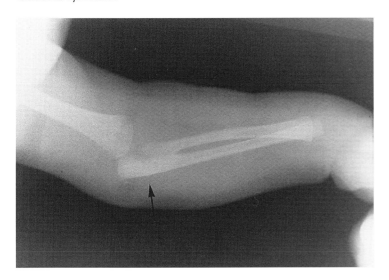

restriction of pronation or supination is detected on examination, it is rarely of clinical importance. A bony prominence is nearly always palpated at the location of dislocation. The diagnosis is established by appropriate radiographs.

Acquired traumatic dislocation of the radial head is the most common condition to be differentiated. The history, the shape of the dislocated radial head, and the shape of the capitellum, are helpful in establishing the type. In a congenital dislocation, the capitellum of the humerus is grossly underdeveloped and the radial head has a rounded or ovoid shape (Figure 6.9). In general, treatment consists of mere observation, unless there is evidence of chronic pain with rotary movements of the elbow in adolescence and puberty. Once skeletal maturation has been achieved, painful dislocations may be dealt with surgically, but only after a conservative program of nonsteroidal anti-inflammatory medications and corticosteroid injections. Attempts to re-establish normal anatomy have usually been exercises in futility, with resulting stiffness being quite common. Attempts to resect the radial head prior to skeletal maturation have resulted in irreparable damage to wrist function. The vast majority of children will evolve into asymptomatic adults with excellent function. Appropriate orthopedic referral after identification is reasonable.

Congenital radio-ulnar synostosis

Congenital radio-ulnar synostosis, or fusion of the proximal ends of the radius and ulna, is an uncommon condition with a hereditary predisposition. Males and females are affected equally, and it occurs bilaterally in well over half of the cases. The fusion of the proximal end of the radius and ulna results in varying degrees of restriction of forearm pronation and supination (Figure 6.10). The usual clinical position is that of mid-pronation or hyperpronation. The diagnosis can be readily established both clinically and radiographically. The functional impairment results from the degree of restricted supination and fixed pronation. Because of the large range of compensatory motion available through the shoulder and the elbow and wrist, unilateral cases usually present with minimal functional disability. Bilateral cases in fixed pronation may occasionally require surgical repositioning of the forearm due to functional disability as a result of the inability to supinate either extremity.

Congenital absence of the radius

Congenital absence of the radius represents a component within the spectrum of congenital amputations of the upper extremity. It has generally been termed the radial "clubhand" in the orthopedic literature. At least 50 percent of the cases are bilateral, and the right side appears to be affected more than the left. Males are affected slightly more frequently than females. The range of clinical abnormality may run the gamut from a slightly hypoplastic radius with a hypoplastic thumb, to a complete absence of the radius and thumb with a rigidly deformed clubhand. Not uncommonly it is associated with systemic disorders; the most worrisome of which are blood dyscrasias and cardiac anomalies (Fanconi's anemia, TAR syndrome, and the Holt–Oram septal defect syndrome). A careful physical examination is essential, because of potential multisystem involvement.

The deformity is readily identifiable at birth, and the diagnosis is easily established by the clinical deformity combined with the radiographic appearance (Figure 6.11). Not only is the hand, wrist, and forearm involved but the elbow joint may also be stiff and contracted. As in all congenital limb absences, the soft tissues are abnormally affected in the hand and forearm. In addition to the muscles and nerves, the ulnar artery may be the only major vascular supply in the forearm and hand.

Figure 6.11. Anteroposterior radiograph demonstrating complete absence of the radius and radial clubhand.

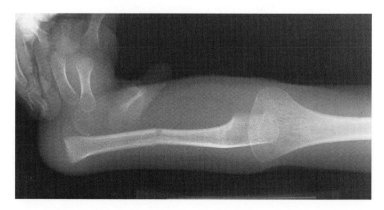

The extent of the functional disability is purely a reflection of unilateral or bilateral involvement. Functional impairment in a bilateral case may be profound and necessitate extensive surgical management. The basic approach to treatment consists of early orthotic management combined with surgical attempts to reposition the wrist and hand on the forearm and maximize the use of functioning digits. The role of the primary care physician is with early diagnosis and appropriate orthopedic referral.

Congenital coxa vara (developmental coxa vara)

Congenital coxa vara is also termed developmental or infantile coxa vara. It is a rare condition characterized by a cartilaginous defect in the femoral neck metaphysis in which a radiolucent line develops in the metaphysis of the proximal femoral neck of the femur attached to the epiphyseal growth plate. The defect is associated with an increasing varus deformity of the proximal femur and limb shortening. The condition affects both males and females. Unilateral involvement is much more common than bilateral involvement.

The etiology of the condition is unknown, although heredity seems to be operative in a number of cases. The etiology of the primary defect seen in radiographic appearance is also unknown, although the influence of weight bearing and chronic slow trauma has been implicated. As the degree of varus increases, the epiphyseal growth plate becomes more vertical and less horizontal. A vicious cycle takes place in which increasing weight bearing forces tend to add to the increasing deformity.

The condition is rarely detected prior to walking, and the child generally presents with a "lurching" type of painless limp. The gait commonly resembles a "duck waddle." The diagnosis is established radiographically by the presence of an inverted "V" triangular piece of metaphyseal bone in the femoral neck adjacent to the growth plate (Figure 6.12). Bilateral congenital coxa vara should cause suspicion of a more generalized skeletal dysplasia. Management of the condition rests with surgical reconstruction of the upper end of the femur to realign the angular deformity (Figure 6.13). The role of the primary care physician is clearly in identification and in appropriate referral.

Congenital pseudoarthrosis of the clavicle

Congenital pseudoarthrosis of the clavicle is a rare condition, presenting at any time from infancy throughout the first decade as a painless mass overlying the mid-portion of the clavicle. Nearly all of the reported cases have occurred on the right side. Because of the routine right-sidedness, it has been postulated that this condition arises in the embryo as a sequela of exaggerated arterial pulsation with secondary pressure on the developing clavicle by the subclavian artery. It is not to be confused with a fracture of the clavicle, which always go on to clinical union in the infant.

Clinically and radiographically, the outer portion of the clavicle appears tilted downward and the shoulder may have the appearance of sitting at a lower level than the opposite side (Figure 6.14). There is a large, rubbery, firm mass overlying the mid-portion of the clavicle that is nontender. Function is not impaired and the deformity results in only cosmetic disability. Union, after modern grafting techniques, has been obtained in some cases. More often than not, surgical attempts to realign and anastomose the clavicular fragments have been mere exercises in futility. Because of the lack of functional impairment, treatment should be directed to the cosmetic deformity alone. Reduction of the volume of the cartilage and bony mass have provided cosmetic improvement. Most cases will not require any treatment.

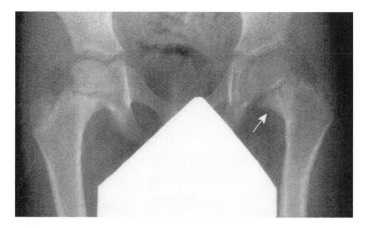

Figure 6.12. Anteroposterior radiograph demonstrating characteristic varus deformity in congenital coxa vara.

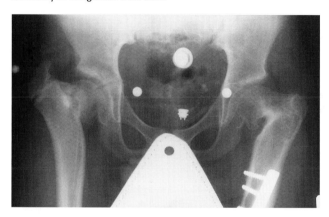

Figure 6.13. Anteroposterior radiograph demonstrating bilateral congenital coxa vara treated by proximal femoral osteotomy.

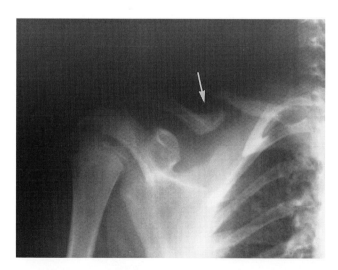

Figure 6.14. Anteroposterior radiograph demonstrating an established congenital pseudo-arthrosis of the clavicle.

Osteogenesis imperfecta

Osteogenesis imperfecta is best thought of as a congenital osteoporosis or osteopenia. It is a connective tissue disorder that results in less bone per unit area and in the formation of a primitive type of "woven bone" that does not ever seem to progress to the much stronger adult form of osteonal bone. There is a great deal of variability in the manifestations of the disease, but there is a basic fragility of bone in all forms that result in fracturing with rather innocuous stresses. The full-blown picture is composed of blue sclera, ligamentous hyperlaxity, abnormal dentinogenesis, excess sweating, easy bruising and fracturing. The fundamental defect in osteogenesis imperfecta is caused by a mutation in type I collagen genes that adversely affect collagen maturation.

Traditionally osteogenesis imperfecta has been separated into two distinct forms: the congenital type and the tarda type. The congenital form is characterized by innumerable fractures at birth and a very poor prognosis with a very high mortality rate secondary to intracranial hemorrhages, or recurrent respiratory infections. In the tarda type, fracturing generally occurs in the first decade of life, and the ensuing deformities are generally not as severe as in the congenital form. There may, however, be numerous fractures and a propensity for the fractures to heal with considerable deformity. Genetically, osteogenesis imperfecta can occur in a dominant form, a recessive form, and even in the form of a spontaneous mutation. Sillence's classification (I–IV) has more recently served to define the congenital and tarda types further and to relate the various clinical findings prognostically (Pearl 6.11).

The diagnosis is established by the clinical stigmata, accompanied by easy fracturing, joint laxity, short stature, and very characteristic radiographic features. The long bones are generally short and slender, with very thin cortices (Figure 6.15). Fractures in various stages of healing are commonly seen.

Pearl 6.11. Sillence classification of osteogenesis imperfecta

Type 1 Blue sclera
  No dentinogenesis defect
Type 2 Lethal
  Blue sclera
  Severe fractures
Type 3 Moderate to severe fracturing
  Dentinogenesis defect
  Mild blue sclera
  Kyphoscoliosis
  Wheelchair
Type 4 Normal sclera
  Moderate fracturing
  No dentinogenesis defect

Figure 6.15. Anteroposterior (a) and lateral (b) radiographs of femur in osteogenesis imperfecta demonstrating marked osteopenia, thin cortices, and previous fractures.

(a) (b)

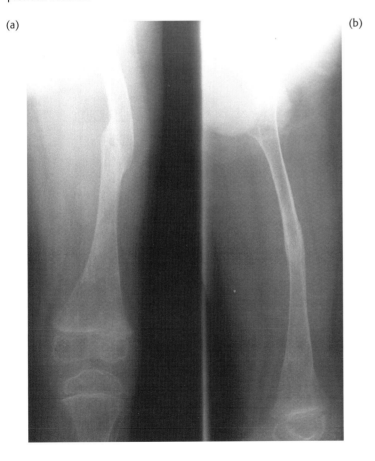

Ossification is often delayed, and the skull may show a very thin calvarium with a mushroom type appearance. The characteristic findings are that of a profound osteoporosis involving all of the bones to a varying degree. Puberty seems to have a stabilizing effect on the frequency of fractures likely as a consequence of hormonal interplay.

From the physician's standpoint the most common condition that needs to be differentiated from osteogenesis imperfecta in the first year of life is the "battered child" syndrome. Scoliosis is quite common and often severe in the first two decades and treatable hearing loss affects many patients in their forties (otosclerosis). Early orthopedic referral is wise once the diagnosis has been established. The orthopedic objectives of treatment are based on the maintenance of present function and the avoidance of further ensuing deformities following fractures in the long bones and joints. In complex diagnostic dilemmas (i.e., child abuse), cellular cultures can be used to confirm the diagnosis. Recent beneficial results with biphosphonate treatment are encouraging but are still early in evaluation.

Neurofibromatosis (Von Recklinghausen's disease)

Neurofibromatosis is a hereditary systemic disorder that is best characterized as a dysplasia of ectodermal and mesodermal tissues. Although mutations can occur, nearly all cases are transmitted by autosomal dominance. The lesions of neurofibromatosis are composed of cells originating from the Schwann cells and the supporting cells. The lesions are manifested both centrally and peripherally, with involvement of the central nervous system, peripheral neurofibromatosis, and characteristic café-au-lait spots. The café-au-lait spots have smooth edges. Six or more with a diameter of 0.5 cm are required for diagnosis. Usually the lesions will tend to be

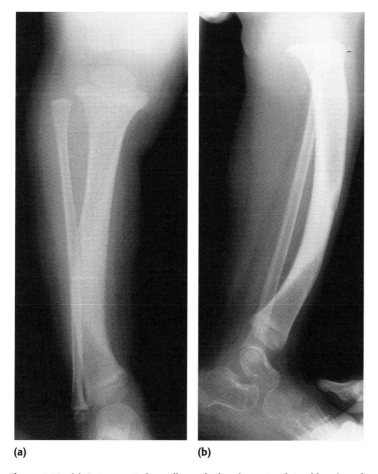

(a)   **(b)**

Figure 6.16. (a) Anteroposterior radiograph showing anterolateral bowing of the tibia associated with neurofibromatosis. (b) Lateral radiograph showing neurofibromatosis producing anterolateral bowing of the tibia.

more prevalent as age increases. The nodules of neurofibromas generally appear during the early second decade. Other stigmata include plexiform neurofibromas, elephantiasis, verrucous hyperplasia, and axillary freckles.

The skeletal findings are quite characteristic and consist of focal gigantism of either an entire limb or a portion of a limb; bowing or pseudoarthrosis, particularly of the tibia, fibula, or forearm bones; and scoliosis, kyphosis, and involvement of the central nervous system in the form of acoustic neuromas and gliomas (Figures 6.16a, b). The scoliosis can often be rapidly progressive. Malignant degeneration occurs in roughly 5–10 percent of the cases. It has been reported that the incidence of malignancy in neurofibromatosis increases with age and may reach an adult level of approximately 20–25 percent.

From the standpoint of the primary care physician, early diagnosis and referral for orthopedic care for the anticipated deformities are advised. Orthopedic management is directed at congenital pseudoarthrosis, scoliosis, and the substantial gigantism with leg length discrepancies.

Fibrous dysplasia

Fibrous dysplasia is a sporadically occurring benign bone dysplasia in which fibro-osseous tissue begins replacing the interior of bones and may also affect extraskeletal sites. It is likely that a failure of conversion woven into lamellar bone exists. It is commonly seen in three different forms: a monostotic (single bone) type, a polyostotic monomelic type in which multiples bones within a given extremity are involved, and a polyostotic generalized form that is commonly associated with precocious puberty (Albright's disease).

Although etiology is unknown, primitive fibrous tissue begins replacing the medullary cavity, expanding the bone from within. The disorder affects both long bones and flat bones, and, not uncommonly, the bones of the skull and face are involved. Clinical findings depend on the location within the bone or bones, and the presence of fracturing. Pain, limping, bowing, and shortening are the usual symptoms encountered. Because of the markedly disturbed and weakened internal architecture of the long bones, fracturing is common. Café-au-lait spots are often seen in association, and have an irregular margin unlike those seen in neurofibromatosis. The presence of sexual precosity is most common in females and is quite striking in nature. Characteristically on standard radiographs the lesions of fibrous dysplasia produce a "ground glass" consistency (Figure 6.17). There is usually cortical erosion from the expansile lesion. Although the location is generally metaphyseal, the lesions tend to spread into the diaphysis, producing expansion of the cortex and increasing deformity. Characteristically a "shepherd's crook" deformity occurs in the upper end of the femur and is quite characteristic of fibrous dysplasia (Figure 6.18). Although the lesions tend to grow and expand during the period of growth, progression is extremely uncommon once skeletal maturation occurs. There is little risk of malignancy, as malignant transformation has been estimated as less than one half of one percent. The diagnosis is established by surgical biopsy.

Appropriate orthopedic referral is indicated once the diagnosis is established. Most patients will develop problems relative to the bony involvement such as angular deformity, scoliosis, and limb length inequality. Pathologic fractures are managed in a conventional orthopedic fashion and healing is to be anticipated.

Hemangiomatosis and lymphangiomatosis

Hemangiomatosis and lymphangiomatosis are hamartomatous lesions of primarily the deep soft tissues that by their presence affect the size, shape, and length of the limbs. The lesions

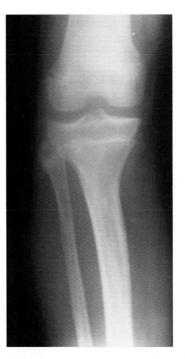

Figure 6.17. Anteroposterior radiograph showing characteristic changes within the tibia and fibula of fibrous dysplasia.

Figure 6.18. Anteroposterior radiograph showing characteristic "shepherd's crook" deformity seen in fibrous dysplasia.

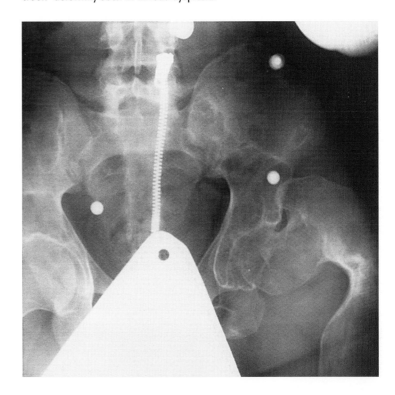

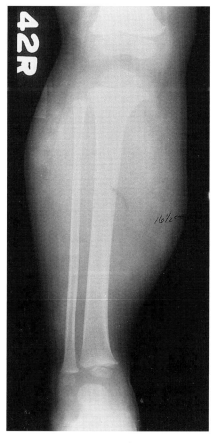

Figure 6.19. Anteroposterior radiograph showing extensive calcification and fusiform enlargement of the soft tissues in hemangiomatosis.

Figure 6.20. Computed tomography images showing markedly enlarged angiomatous lesions in the soft tissue with calcification in hemangiomatosis.

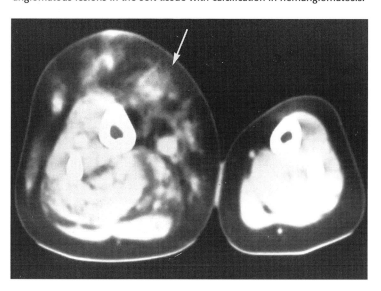

may consist primarily of hemangiomatous type tissue, or of tortuous dilated lymphatic channels, most likely arising from a common cellular origin (Figures 6.19 & 6.20).

Clinically, patients so affected may present with pain in the extremity, but more usually as a result of regional gigantism, leg length discrepancy, and limb deformity. Intramuscular hemangiomas are common and can be painful. Well defined, rounded calcifications (pheboliths) may be seen on radiographs. In more involved cases an entire limb or an entire portion of the body may be involved with these slowly enlarging lesions. The clinical manifestations usually require a combination of plastic surgery and orthopedic surgery. Appropriate recognition should result in appropriate referral.

Osteochondroma (osteochondromatosis)

The basic lesion of osteochondroma or osteochondromatosis is a benign cartilage capped protrusion of osseous tissue arising from the surface of bone. The cortex of the bone is continuous with the osteochondroma and the medullary canal extends directly into the base of the lesion. Although the lesion tends to resemble a neoplasm, it is likely a disturbance in enchondral growth, both in location and direction. It is best conceived as the body's attempt to form an additional bone in an abnormal location. It is likely that these lesions arise as an aberration in the direction of growth within the peripheral portion of the epiphyseal growth plate, producing a bone that then proceeds to grow along the path of least resistance. The lesions seen in the solitary form of osteochondroma and in multiple form of osteochondromatosis (multiple hereditary exostosis) are histologically identical in nature. The most common location for a solitary osteochondroma is the distal end of the femur and the proximal end of the tibia and humerus. Clinically the lesion is recognized as a hard, non-mobile mass that is usually non-painful. Occasionally irritation of surrounding tissues will produce a localized bursitis or tendonitis. Radiographic appearance is characteristic, with a bony protuberance with the same bony texture as the adjacent bony tissue from which it arises (Figure 6.21). It also appears quite mature in its periphery. The lesions have different forms and shapes that are either classified as sessile (cauliflower-like), or pedunculated (stalk-like). They may occur in flat bones but are much more common in long bones. Surgical exploration is indicated in both solitary and multiple osteochondroma for pain, or for the very rare case that shows suspicious signs of malignancy on radiography.

The multiple form (multiple hereditary exostosis) is usually inherited in an autosomal dominant fashion. It is routinely associated with shortness of stature, and the presence of multiple lesions throughout nearly all of the long bones and many of the flat bones (Figure 6.22). It is slightly more common in males and is not associated with any reduction in life span. The clinical findings encompass all of those noted with solitary osteochondromas and include shortness of stature, and a characteristic deviation of the wrist toward the ulnar side, a reflection of retarded growth of the distal ulna. Not uncommonly, a valgus deformity of the ankle may develop, due to disproportionate growth between the tibia and fibula secondary to involvement by the lesions. The upper end of the femur develops a valgoverted (valgus-anteversion) type of malalignment. Indications for surgery are identical with solitary osteochondroma. Sarcomatous transformation is uncommon and rates have been published ranging from less than one percent to 10 percent. It is more likely that the incidence of malignancy is around one percent at the most. Lesions that continue to grow past puberty or are painful in the skeletally mature should be suspected to be malignant. Diagnosis is important from the primary care standpoint and that appropriate

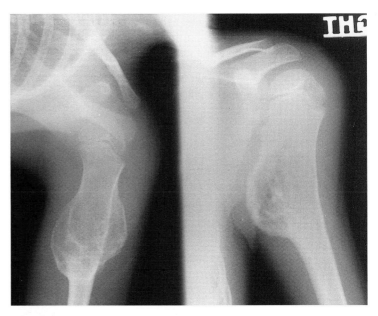

Figure 6.21. Large sessile osteochondroma of the proximal humerus.

Figure 6.22. Anteroposterior radiograph showing multiple osteochondromatosis.

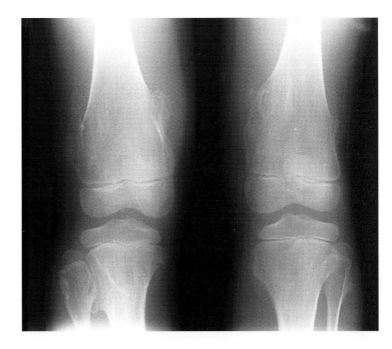

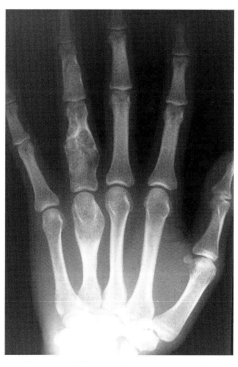

Figure 6.23. Anteroposterior radiograph of the hand demonstrating a large enchondroma involving proximal phalanx fourth digit.

Figure 6.24. Anteroposterior radiograph of the proximal humerus demonstrating enchondromatous involvement.

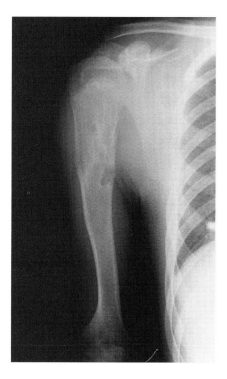

orthopedic referral is made for the above-mentioned clinical factors.

Enchondroma and enchondromatosis (Ollier's disease)

Solitary enchondroma and multiple enchondromatosis bear the same relationship to each other as do osteochondroma to osteochondromatosis. Solitary enchondromas occur equally in males and females, and are generally seen in the latter half of the first decade onward into adult life. The cartilaginous lesions lie within the substance of the medullary system of the limb bones, with a high predilection for involvement of the phalanges (Figure 6.23) and metacarpals and metatarsals. Occasionally lesions are also seen in the humerus and femur (Figure 6.24). Although the lesions are generally detected on routine evaluation of a limb for other problems, pathologic fractures or increasing deformity are the usual cause of symptomatology. In addition to the local signs of fracture the involved bone is usually expanded in nature and misshapen due to the intraosseous lesion. Malignant transformation of a solitary enchondroma in the distal extremities is extremely rare, although somewhat higher in long tubular bones. The exact incidence of malignant transformation is unknown, although it is felt to be extremely uncommon. Appropriate identification by the primary care physician and orthopedic referral is indicated as some of these lesions will require curettage and bone grafting (more central axial lesions need periodic radiographic observation).

Multiple enchondromatosis is a very rare condition in which there is a substantial proliferation of cartilage cells originating within the bone substance itself and also from the periosteum. The involvement may be of a single extremity, a portion of the extremity, or multiple extremities (Figure 6.25). In general, the long bones are shortened, bowed, and broadened. Commonly, near the joints, the enlargements resemble large bulbous excrescences producing considerable cosmetic deformity. Leg length discrepancies are common in the multiple form. The association of multiple enchondromatosis and multiple hemangiomas has been termed *Maffucci's syndrome*. Diagnosis is established by the clinical picture coupled with characteristic radiographs. There appears to be an increased incidence of malignant transformation in adult life with the exact incidence being unknown. Orthopedic management generally involves the treatment of limb length inequality, fracture care, and progressive follow-up of the lesions as to their malignant potential. Appropriate diagnosis and referral from the primary care standpoint is indicated.

Unicameral bone cyst

Unicameral bone cyst is a single cavity lined with a thin membrane and usually containing straw-colored fluid. Occasionally there may be little else but an empty cavity. It is slightly more common in males, and most commonly is seen in the upper end of the humeral metaphysis. Involvement of the femur and humerus accounts for well over three-quarters of all reported cases (Figure 6.26). The remainder of the cases are well distributed throughout the body. Although there have been many hypotheses as to the etiology of these cysts, the most common currently accepted etiology is based on the theory of localized venous obstruction and subsequent intramedullary erosion. The closer the proximity of the cyst to the physis, and presence of fluid (blood) under pressure with the cyst, the greater the chance of recurrence after any type of treatment.

It is recommended that patients with bone cysts be referred to the orthopedic surgeon for continuing management. Orthopedic treatment currently consists initially of fenestration of the lesion, infiltration with

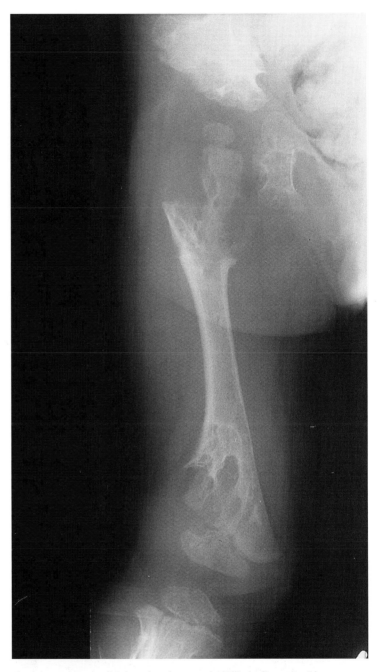

Figure 6.25. Generalized enchondromatosis (Ollier's disease) with extensive involvement of the femur.

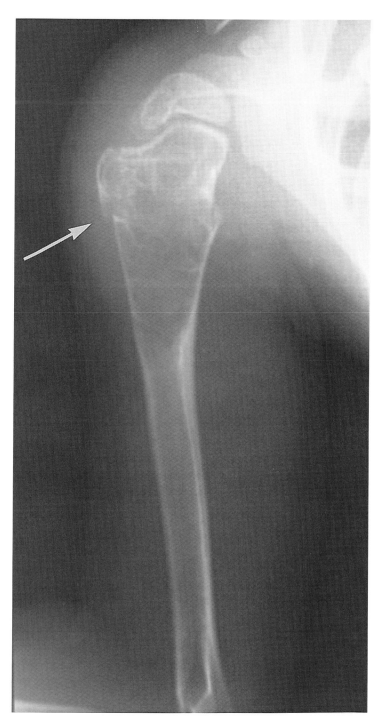

Figure 6.26. Anteroposterior radiograph demonstrating a pathologic fracture through a large unicameral bone cyst.

corticosteroids or other chemical compounds, incision, curettage and bone grafting for failures, and commonly simple periodic observation. The lesions tend to disappear eventually with skeletal maturity and are extremely uncommon in adulthood.

Aneurysmal bone cyst

An aneurysmal bone cyst is composed of vascular channels that contain blood or serosanguineous fluid. The vascular channels do not resemble human blood vessels. The etiology is unknown. It is most commonly seen in the latter part of the first decade, and particularly in the early and mid-portions of the second decade. At least half of the cases have been reported in the long bones of the limbs, although the axial skeleton is not uncommonly involved, particularly the vertebra.

Usually the lesion is detected in a routine radiograph for another problem. The most common complaints are of aching pain, and only rarely, a bony prominence. Inasmuch as the lesion weakens the surrounding bone, a fracture may be the initial sign of a problem. The diagnosis is established by both radiographic appearance and histologic evidence on biopsy (Figure 6.27). Orthopedic management consists of surgical extirpation of the lesion accompanied by appropriate replacement with bone grafting. Aggressive lesions may require widespread resections and perhaps even the use of allografts. These lesions are far more aggressive than unicameral bone cysts and a relatively high recurrence rate is to be expected. Diagnosis should be accompanied by appropriate orthopedic referral.

Non-ossifying fibroma (metaphyseal fibrous defect)

Non-ossifying fibroma is a developmental fibrous defect of bone in which bundles of fibrous connective tissue replace normal bone within either the cortex of the bone or the cancellous bone. The lesions are clearly benign. There is a blend in terminology between metaphyseal fibrous defects of bone and nonossifying fibroma, but the behavior is clinically similar and the histology is identical. The vast majority of the lesions lie within the distal metaphysis of the femur, and are usually cortical in nature. The next most common bone affected in a much smaller percentage of cases is the tibia. It is usually discovered during the first decade of life and is generally asymptomatic, unless a subsequent pathologic fracture ensues.

The radiographic appearance of these lesions is rather distinctive. The lesion is radiolucent and eccentrically placed, usually lying within the cortex of the metaphysis of a long bone, with a well-defined sclerotic border (Figures 6.28a, b). A "soap bubble" type of appearance is characteristic. The lesions are clearly radiographically benign, and orthopedic management is indicated for those lesions presenting with a prior pathologic fracture or in which the defect size is of such magnitude as to warrant curettage and bone grafting to prevent additional fracturing. Smaller lesions, which are identified on examination for other diseases, require only periodic observation. The lesions are believed to spontaneously resolve with skeletal maturation. The role of the primary care physician is for appropriate identification and consultation and / or referral.

Osteoid osteoma

Osteoid osteoma is a benign reactive lesion of bone characterized by a central active nidus that is composed of a very highly vascular connective tissue centrum and surrounded by dense reactive bone. Although it has been traditionally taught that the lesions are non-neoplastic, non-inflammatory, or infectious, the behavior strongly mimics that of a localized inflammatory process. The lesion

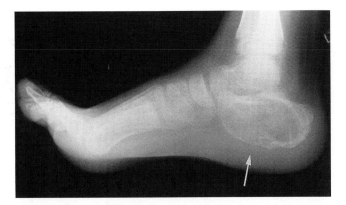

Figure 6.27. Lateral radiograph of the foot demonstrating a large aneurysmal bone cyst within the calcaneus.

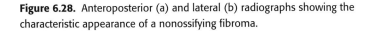

Figure 6.28. Anteroposterior (a) and lateral (b) radiographs showing the characteristic appearance of a nonossifying fibroma.

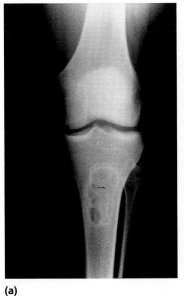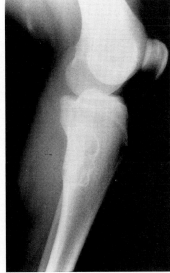

(a)   **(b)**

(a)

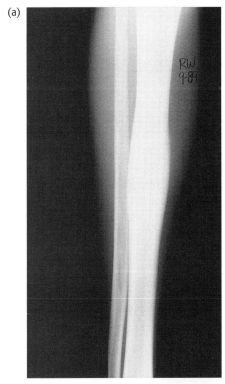

(b)

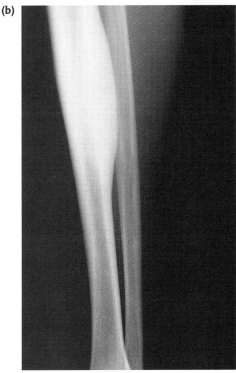

Figure 6.29. Anteroposterior (a) and lateral (b) radiographs of the tibia showing fusiform expansion and cortical thickening associated with osteoid osteoma.

clinically behaves like a low-grade localized infection of bone, which does not result in an abscess, or the more serious sequelae of other types of infection. It is likely that the true etiology will be debated for many years, but the condition is generally self-limiting, occurs more commonly in males, and most commonly affects a single bone.

The clinical findings are usually characteristic, although may also be subtle in nature. Pain is the most significant complaint, and very commonly occurs in the evening or at night, awakening the patient from sleep. If the lesion is sufficiently superficial in location, localized tenderness may be present, and there may even be some local deformation from the reactive bone in the region of the lesion. When present in the spine, painful scoliosis may occur. An antalgic gait (painful limp) may be present in lower extremity involvement. Commonly the radiographic appearance is quite typical and consists of a central radiolucent nidus up to 1 cm in size surrounded by dense sclerotic bone adjacent to the nidus (Figures 6.29a, b). The bony reaction can be quite substantial and usually far more extensive than the central nidus. Standard tomograms and particularly thin cut computed tomography (2–3 mm) images are quite helpful (Figure 6.30). Bone imaging is an important adjunct and very helpful in defining the exact location. It is common for the disease to run its course within a five-year period whether treated or untreated. Salicylates and other anti-inflammatories have been found to be quite effective in ameliorating the symptoms, although it may take upwards of two to three years of treatment time. Continuing discomfort has often necessitated localized en bloc excision of the lesion, and recently developed computerized tomographic directed needle biopsy has been quite successful without necessitating removal of excessive amounts of bony tissue. Irradiation and chemotherapy have not been found to be of value. The role of the primary care physician consists of diagnosis, occasionally medication treatment and appropriate orthopedic referral.

Histiocytosis X

Histiocytosis X is a syndrome best characterized by the presence of granulomatous lesions composed of histiocytes that represent a spectrum of conditions. The term includes Letterer–Siwe disease, Hand–Schuller–Christian disease, and eosinophilic granuloma of bone. Letterer–Siwe disease is the acute disseminated progressive life-threatening form of this histiocytosis, with both visceral and bony involvement. Hand–Schuller–Christian disease is the more chronic disseminated form of histiocytosis X, with minimal or moderate visceral involvement, and bone involvement. The diagnosis and management of these two conditions will be left for more appropriate medical textbooks. Eosinophilic granuloma of bone is a histiocytic granuloma that affects both the flat and long bones, is more common in males than females, and is most commonly seen in the latter portion of the first decade. The most common location for involvement is the skull, with the next most common site being the femur. Involvement of nearly every bone has been described.

The most common presenting symptom is localized pain in the area of bone involvement. Localized swelling is common, and localized tenderness may be present. The expansile nature of the lesion may weaken the surrounding bone and lead to fracture. Characteristically the radiographic appearance is that of a radiolucent "punched out" appearance with very little, if any, bony reaction to the lesion unless a fracture is present. There is often great variability in radiographic presentation. A skeletal survey is recommended in nearly all cases to evaluate a more systemic distribution. Other characteristics of a benign bone lesion are generally present. Progressive involvement of the skull to an advanced degree gives the

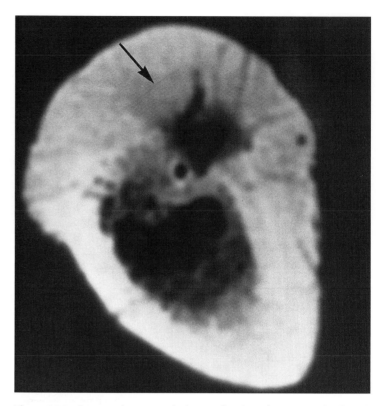

Figure 6.30. Computed tomography image showing a large cortical nidus of osteoid osteoma.

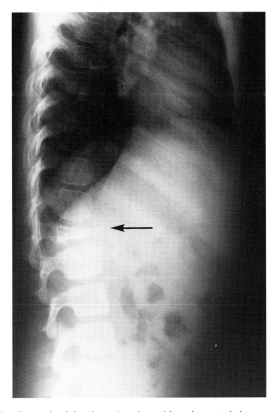

Figure 6.31. Lateral radiograph of the thoracic spine with a characteristic "coin-shaped" vertebrae associated with vertebra plana (eosinophilic granuloma).

Figure 6.32. Lateral cervical radiograph demonstrating vertebra plana seen in eosinophilic granuloma.

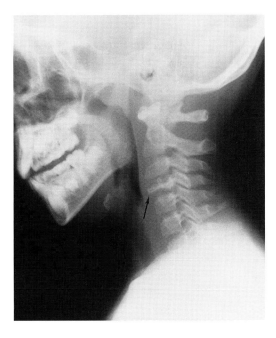

appearance known as the "geographic" skull. Involvement of the vertebra can produce a lesion known as *verterbra plana* (Figure 6.31). In the vertebra, the lesion produces intraosseous collapse, but does not appear to affect the adjacent disc spaces ("coin-shaped" vertebra) (Figure 6.32). In the long bones, the lesions involve the diaphysis as well as the metaphysis and produce their damage by expansion and erosion from within. A radiographic skeletal survey is indicated, and generally provides more information than radionuclide imaging, as many of the lesions are "cold" on scanning. Treatment consists of closed or open biopsy, and histologic documentation of the nature of the lesion.

Eosinophilic granuloma of bone is a benign lesion that generally will undergo spontaneous healing, whether treated or untreated. Decisions to proceed with wide curettage and grafting, intralesional injection of steroids, or simple biopsy and observation, are arrived at by the location within the bone and the subsequent potential damage from the lesion (fracture potential). It is important for the primary care physician to be aware of this lesion, and with appropriate radiographic and histologic diagnosis, proceed to orthopedic referral.

Malignant soft tissue and bone lesions

The basic characteristic of malignant soft tissue lesions is an enlarging, firm, painful mass. Malignant bone lesions are often painful in contrast to benign processes. Persistent growth and increasing firmness of a soft tissue mass are hallmarks of malignancy. Lesions deep to the fascia and greater than 5 cm deserve particular attention. Night pain, loss of motion, and radiographic image evidence of a soft tissue component to a bone lesion increase the index of suspicion for malignancy. Standard radiographic examination of the affected portion of the body is always indicated. If a diagnosis cannot be established on clinical assessment and standard radiographs, magnetic resonance imaging is almost always the best means of evaluation. Computed tomography scanning and bone scanning are of little use in soft tissue malignancies. Ultrasonography may be preferable to magnetic resonance imaging in popliteal soft tissue masses for popliteal cysts.

For suspicious lesions, adequate biopsy material is necessary. A core biopsy or open biopsy is the procedure of choice for nearly all lesions and should, if at all possible, be performed by the treating surgeon. An experienced pathologist is essential. If standard radiographs cannot establish the diagnosis of a bone lesion, whole body scanning can be helpful to evaluate activity. Increased activity on bone scan does not necessarily imply malignancy. Multicentric or metastatic lesions may be manifest on scanning. "Cold scans" generally indicate a benign nature. Skeletal surveys should be considered in evaluating malignant tumors.

Computed tomography scanning provides an excellent view of bone but is of less value for soft tissues. Computed tomography scanning is particularly valuable in evaluating benign bone lesions that may be at risk for fracturing. Magnetic resonance imaging is particularly helpful for the extent of soft tissue involvement and bone marrow involvement. Core biopsy and particularly open biopsy are essential in suspected malignancy to provide adequate tissue for examination.

Rhabdomyosarcoma

Rhabdomyosarcoma is the most common soft tissue sarcoma in childhood. The tumors are highly aggressive and require aggressive treatment. Tumor staging includes regional lymph node biopsy, chest/ abdominal/ pelvic computed tomography scanning and a bone marrow aspiration. Local therapy consists of complete surgical excision with adjunctive radiation therapy added if there is incomplete excision of the lesion. Rhabdomyosarcomas are

Figure 6.33. Calcification within a synovial sarcoma.

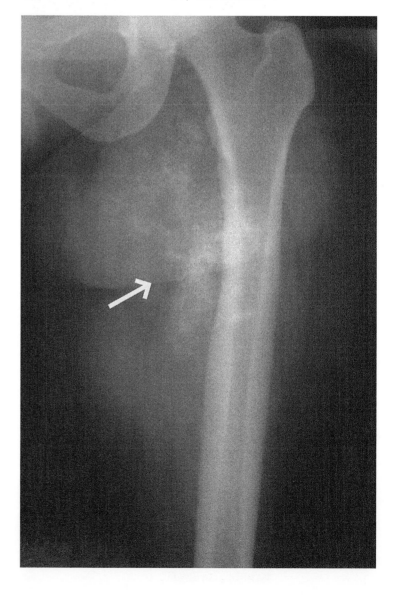

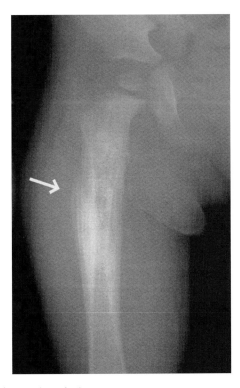

Figure 6.34. "Onion-skin" changes in Ewing's sarcoma.

Figure 6.35. "Sunburst" pattern in osteosarcoma.

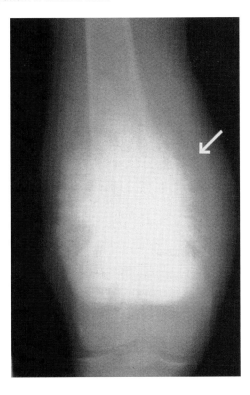

one of the only soft tissue sarcomas routinely treated with chemotherapy. A 50–70 percent, three-year survival rates can be currently expected when there is no evidence of metastatic disease at presentation.

Synovial sarcoma

Synovial sarcomas are soft tissue sarcomas that occur near joints but do not typically arise from joints. It is the most common soft tissue sarcoma in older adolescents and younger adults. Radiographs may demonstrate calcification (up to 40 percent) (Figure 6.33). Magnetic resonance imaging evaluation is essential but cannot differentiate one soft tissue tumor from another. Surgical wide excision with negative margins is essential for all soft tissue sarcomas. Radiation therapy is often necessary for high-grade lesions (histologic) to diminish recurrences. Chemotherapy is currently being investigated but is as yet of unproved value. Five-year survival rates of up to 80 percent can currently be expected with appropriate treatment.

Ewing's sarcoma

Ewing's sarcoma is a malignant permeative diaphyseal lesion with indistinct borders and accompanied by an aggressive periosteal reaction ("onion-skinning") (Figure 6.34). Patients almost always present with pain and a soft tissue mass. Often, patients have fevers, chills, and diaphoresis that can mimic infection. Chest CT scanning, bone scanning, and bone marrow aspiration should be performed in search of metastatic disease. All patients will require multi-drug chemotherapy. Local involvement dictates wide margin surgical extirpation almost always with limb salvage. Radiation therapy, once the preferred mode of treatment, is currently reserved for unresectable disease or incomplete surgery. Currently three-year survival rates of approximately 60 percent can be expected with appropriate treatment.

Osteosarcoma

Osteosarcoma is most commonly seen during adolescence or early adulthood. Pain and limp are typical. The classic radiographic feature is a metaphyseal bone-forming lesion with a "sunburst" periosteal reaction (Figure 6.35). Computed tomography scanning of the chest is mandatory to evaluate metastatic disease. Following biopsy, wide local surgery is indicated followed by chemotherapy. Limb salvage procedures can be performed except with extensive local disease. Radiation therapy does not play a role routinely. With modern surgery and chemotherapy, the five-year survival rates are approximately 80–85 percent (Pearls 6.12, 6.13).

Pearl 6.12. Indications for orthopedic referral

Large, deeply located lesions
Subfascial lesions >5 cm
or
Increase in size or firmness
Painful masses
Uncertain diagnosis of a bone lesion after
    radiographs and magnetic resonance
    imaging
Painful benign lesions

Pearl 6.13. Suspicious radiographic evidence for bone malignancy

Cortical disruption
Periosteal reaction ("onion-skinning",
    "sunburst")
Soft tissue mass
Extensive bone destruction

Chapter 7

Genetic disorders of the musculoskeletal system

General considerations

The genetic disorders of the musculoskeletal system are reflected in a heterogeneous group of conditions generally referred to as skeletal dysplasias. Most, but not all, result in significant shortness of stature (dwarfism), most are rare but phenotypic varieties are numerous (roughly 200–300 different types) and are generally accompanied by disproportionate short stature. Dwarfism is commonly characterized by an adult height of 1.2 m (c. 4′ 10″) or below. The term disproportionate dwarfism applies to those individuals whose relative shortening is different between the trunk and extremities and unequal often within the extremities themselves. In proportionate short stature, the relative degree of shortness equally affects the trunk and extremities and portions of the extremities.

The term rhizomelic dwarfism infers that the proximal segments (humerus and femur) are disproportionately shorter than the middle segments (radius–ulna and tibia–fibula) and the distal segments (wrists–hands and ankles–feet). The term mesomelia refers to disproportionate shortness in which the middle segments (radius–ulna and tibia–fibula) are shorter than their counterparts in the proximal and distal regions. The term acromelia refers to greater distal shortening (wrists–hands and ankles–feet) relative to the more proximal portions. Micromelia simply describes shortness of a limb.

The term dysplasia relates to those conditions affecting growing bone and cartilage where the primary defect is intrinsic to bone. Nearly all these conditions are genetically determined and result in primary bone and cartilage defects from their inception. Dysostosis refers to those affectations of bone and cartilage in which the bone and cartilage form normally initially, and are secondarily affected by errors in the remodeling and reshaping process. Usually individual bones are affected rather than a generalized disorder. Dystrophy refers to those disorders of bone and cartilage in which the bone is normal in early formation and then is secondarily affected by extrinsic factors such as hormonal disturbances and metabolic diseases. The diagnosis of a skeletal dysplasia may be extremely easy for relatively severe cases or much more difficult in cases of less severe phenotypic expression.

The identification of specific genes, mutations, and genotype–phenotype relationships has dramatically augmented our accuracy in establishing specific diagnoses. Retarded growth may be due to failure of almost any organ system, however body proportions are usually retained unless the primary pathology involves the genetic factors controlling skeletal growth and maturation. Mutations of genes which produce the proteins essential for skeletal integrity result in qualitative and quantitative abnormalities of these proteins (e.g., structural proteins and enzymes). These genetic mutations result in defects characterized by altered growth, strength, or maturity of the connective tissue and leads to disproportionate growth of body parts. Of the many genetic disorders of the musculoskeletal system, only a few of the more common disorders will be discussed in this chapter.

Achondroplasia

Achondroplasia is the most common form of skeletal dysplasia producing dwarfism, and

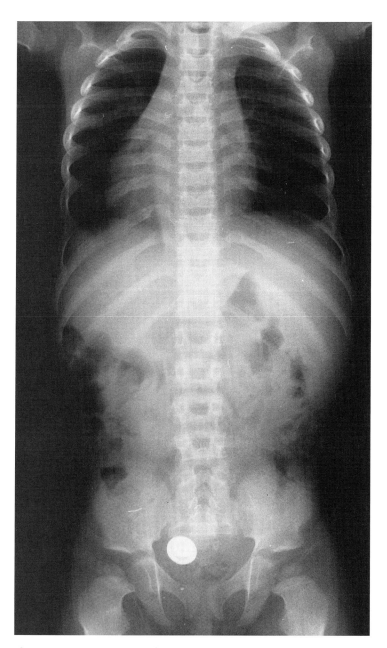

Figure 7.1. Anteroposterior radiograph of the thoracolumbar spine showing reduced interpedicular distance in the lower lumbar spine, squared acetabulae, and the characteristic pelvic inlet (champagne glass) seen in achondroplasia.

represents the classic disorder of enchondral bone formation. It is genetically and clinically a homogeneous disorder with remarkably consistent physical and radiographic findings. More than 98 percent of patients with achondroplasia have the same single nucleotide mutation in the fibroblast growth factor receptor 3 (FGFR3) gene. A person with achondroplasia who has a partner with normal stature has a 50 percent risk in every pregnancy of having a child with achondroplasia. Intramembranous bone formation proceeds quite normally. An achondroplastic dwarf is the classic example of a rhizomelic disorder (proximal long bones shorter than distal). Patients exhibit clinically short-limbed dwarfism, prominent forehead, low flattened nasal bridge, bowing of the lower extremities, lumbar lordosis, narrowed cervical and lumbar spinal canal with spinal canal stenosis, and potential spinal cord and nerve root impingement. Although roughly 90 percent of all achondroplasia appears sporadically as a spontaneous mutation, it is inherited as an autosomal dominant. Natural selection likely has resulted in its sporadic appearance.

The radiographic features of this condition are striking and diagnostic, even in utero. The most striking radiographic changes are the narrowing of the interpedicular distance of the lumbar spine (Figure 7.1), squared acetabulum, ball and socket epiphyses (Figure 7.2), "trident" hand, sharp sciatic notch with markedly reduced iliac height, and severe genu varum. Cervical spine stenosis can result in death in the first year of life if unrecognized. Thin cut computed tomography scanning or magnetic resonance imaging is very useful in defining the extent of cervical canal stenosis and early recognition should be accompanied by surgical decompression.

In general, neither life span nor cognitive ability are affected by this condition, and problems later in life generally relate to chronic sciatica and lumbar disc disease, spinal stenosis, and angular deformities. Primary care physicians should have an awareness of the condition and provide for appropriate orthopedic or skeletal dysplasia clinic referral if deformities become manifest.

Mucopolysaccharidoses

The mucopolysaccharidoses constitute the largest group of lysosomal storage diseases in humans. Although rare in clinical practice, they are common enough to be confused with other forms of short stature, particularly achondroplasia. All of the six commonly recognized types of mucopolysaccharidoses have in common the failure of lysosomal enzymes to fully break down intracellular compounds, with the resultant accumulation of mucopolysaccharides in abnormal quantities within the cell. The mucopolysaccharides involved in these conditions are active in skeletal growth and development and are composed of heparan sulfate, dermatan sulfate, and keratan sulfate. Abnormal intracellular accumulation of these mucopolysaccharides results in defective growth and development of the skull, ribs, vertebral bodies, pelvis, and long bones, as well as the bones of the hands and feet. These disorders are generally not recognizable at birth, and usually make their appearance in the first or second year of life.

As a group, mucopolysaccharidoses are caused by deficiencies of enzymes in the degradation pathway of proteoglycans. Mucopolysaccharidosis II (Hunter syndrome) is X-linked. All others are autosomal recessive. Accumulations of proteoglycans result in progressive multiorgan tissue damage. This accumulation of proteoglycans may involve bone, cartilage, skin, airways, and the cardiovascular system. Types I, II, and IV will frequently involve the musculoskeletal system. Phenotype analysis often provides a diagnostic clue, but biochemical testing (excess excretion of urinary mucopolysaccharides) is the most common method for diagnosis. Type I mucopolysaccharidosis (Hurler syndrome) is characterized by coarse facial features, macrocephaly, corneal clouding, and mental

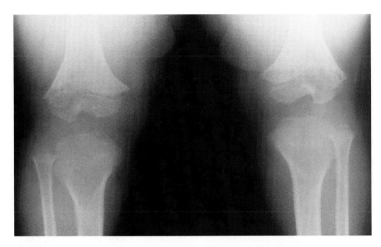

Figure 7.2. Anteroposterior radiographs of the knees demonstrating ball and socket distal femoral epiphysis seen in achondroplasia.

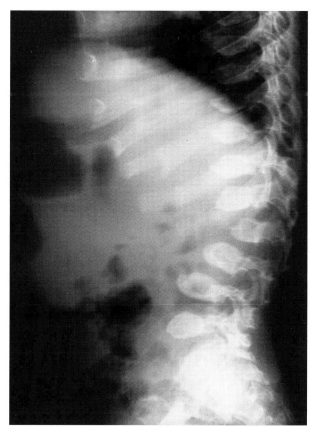

Figure 7.3. Lateral radiograph of the thoracolumbar spine showing characteristic anterior and inferior vertebral beaking seen commonly in the mucopolysaccharidoses.

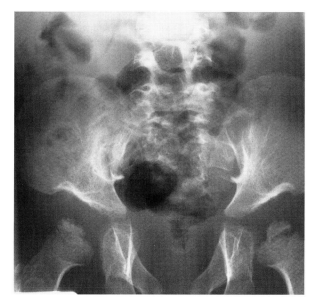

Figure 7.4. Anteroposterior radiograph of the pelvis demonstrating dysplastic changes in the acetabulum with femoral head subluxation seen in mucopolysaccharidoses.

retardation. Hepatosplenomegaly is frequent. Affected individuals have a short, segmented thoracolumbar kyphoscoliosis (gibbus) (Figure 7.3). The long bones are generally thick, short, and misshapen and the joints are often stiff.

The radiographic features of the disorder are impressive and consist of sharp-angled kyphosis at the thoracolumbar level, significant genu valgum, hip dysplasia and subluxation, and commonly, dislocation (Figure 7.4). The pelvic inlet is shaped like a "port wine glass" and the vertebrae often demonstrate anterior–inferior "beaking." The sella turcica is "J"-shaped, and the ribs tend to be shaped like a "canoe paddle." The hands have shortened metacarpals that resemble a "sugar loaf" with "bullet-shaped" phalanges and proximal tapering of the base of the metacarpals, particularly the fifth metacarpal (Figure 7.5). The vast majority of affected children, rarely survive the middle of the second decade.

In type II (Hunter syndrome), there is no thoracolumbar gibbus. It is X-linked recessive occurring exclusively in males. There is no clouding of the cornea, and there is minimal to moderate mental retardation as distinguishing features in both type I and type II mucopolysaccharidoses. There is an increased amount of dermatan and heparan sulfate in the urine.

In type IV (Morquio's–Brailsford syndrome), the condition is characterized by a number of musculoskeletal features. Affected individuals demonstrate a disproportionately short trunk type of dwarfism with marked genu valgum (knock-knees), pectus carinatum (pigeon breast), waddling gait with severely pronated feet, and laxity of most joints, but stiffness of the larger joints. There is protrusion of the lower face with a broad jaw and a short neck. Kyphoscoliosis is commonly seen and may be severe and progressive. There are significant dental abnormalities including enamel hypoplasia. Intelligence is generally normal, and fine corneal deposits are commonly seen.

The radiographic changes most commonly encountered are hypoplasia of the odontoid with increased instability of the atlantoaxial junction that can result in severe cord compression, weakness, and paralysis. There is usually anterior "beaking" of the vertebra. Type IV is characterized by the excretion of abnormal amounts of keratan sulfate in urine. Morbidity is related to cord compression from the upper cervical instability and kyphoscoliosis and occasionally hip degeneration.

The diagnosis rests with the combination of clinical and radiographic features, combined with a determination by either skin fibroblast cultures and/ or urine studies for the appropriate enzyme (Pearls 7.1, 7.2). The role of the primary care physician rests in establishing the appropriate diagnosis. The natural history varies individually throughout the types of mucopolysaccharidoses, and the reader should refer to appropriate medical texts. In general, orthopedic management consists of treatment for accompanying kyphoscoliosis, cervical spine instability, hip dysplasia/ dislocation, and angular deformities of the long bones.

Down syndrome

Down syndrome or trisomy 21 is the most common chromosome abnormality in humans and is accompanied by several disorders of the musculoskeletal system. Trisomy for chromosome 21 is the basic genetic defect. Generalized hypotonia and marked ligamentous laxity is present routinely. There is a generalized retardation of growth with most adult males reaching an average height of 1.5 m (*c*. 5′ 1″) and most females reach 1.2 m (*c*. 4′ 9″). Short phalanges and metacarpals produce a broad, short hand, and hypoplasia of the middle phalanx of the fifth finger causes clinodactyly. Nearly half of these patients have a "simian crease." The feet often show a wide gap between the first and second toes and a characteristic corresponding plantar "furrow" (cleft). Forty percent of patients have cardiac anomalies and all have orthopedic abnormalities.

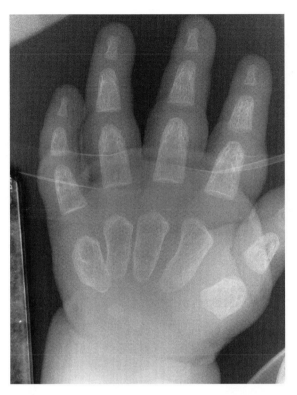

Figure 7.5. Anteroposterior hand radiograph showing "sugar loaf" metacarpals and "bullet-shaped" phalanges seen in mucopolysaccharidoses.

Pearl 7.1. Types of mucopolysaccharidoses

I	H-Hurler
I	S-Scheie
II	Hunter
III	San Filippo
IV	Morquio's–Brailsford
V	Maroteaux and Lamy
VI	SLY

Pearl 7.2. Abnormal mucopolysaccharide accumulations

I	H-dermatan sulfate heparan sulfate
I	S-dermatan sulfate heparan sulfate
II	Dermatan sulfate heparan sulfate
III	Heparan sulfate
IV	Keratan sulfate
V	Dermatan sulfate
VI	Chondroitin sulfate
VII	Dermatan sulfate heparan sulfate

Walking, like other motor development, is delayed and is characterized by a shuffling, broad-based, waddling gait with the lower extremities held in external rotation. The cervical spine may be a source of disability and death in children and young adults with Down syndrome. Compression of the spinal cord may lead to a wide spectrum of neurologic signs and symptoms. Thoracolumbar scoliosis may be present. Often times the hips are hypermobile and occasionally are unstable or dislocated. Likewise, profound ligamentous laxity results in patellar instability with lateral subluxation and dislocation. Almost all affected individuals have a severe flexible flatfoot. True clubfeet can be seen in association with Down syndrome and roughly 90 percent or more of patients will have a metatarsus primus varus or medial deviation of the first toe metatarsal. Radiographically the pelvis is flattened, particularly at the lower edges of the ilium. There is a shallow acetabular roof with widening and flaring of the iliac "wings", and the iliae have the appearance of "elephant ears." Overall morbidity in Down syndrome is generally related to the severity of the cardiac defects and the accompanying dimension of the orthopedic disabilities. Collision sports should probably be avoided due to the potential of upper cervical instability.

Marfan syndrome and homocystinuria

Marfan syndrome is an autosomal dominant connective tissue disorder caused by mutations in the fibrillin (FBN1) gene located on chromosome 15. The diagnosis remains dependent upon clinical findings. The principal manifestations of this disorder are found in the skeletal system, cardiovascular system, and the eye. Marfan syndrome is characterized by tall stature, particularly with elongation of the distal segments of the limbs. This disproportionate growth of the limbs produces a reduced upper segment to lower segment ratio and a span that is greater than the height.

The term dolichostenomelia refers to these long, slender limb bones. Arachnodactyly is a term that has been applied to the long, spindly fingers and toes. Weakness and redundancy of joint capsule and ligaments and tendons may result in joint hypermobility, patellar subluxation, hip dislocation, hyperpronated flat feet (flexible flatfeet), scoliosis, and kyphoscoliosis. Overgrowth or undergrowth of the ribs and sternum commonly produces pectus carinatum or pectus excavatum.

The connective tissue defects result in an evolving pattern of cardiovascular manifestations. Weakness of the aortic wall frequently results in progressive dilatation of the aortic root that may ultimately produce an aneurysm of the ascending aorta. This aortic dilatation may be the prelude to a potentially fatal dissecting aortic aneurysm. The chief ocular consequence of Marfan syndrome is ectopia lentis. The lens displacement is typically upward. Other ophthalmologic findings include myopia, glaucoma, and retinal detachment.

Homocystinuria shares some of the phenotypic characteristics seen in Marfan syndrome. In contrast to Marfan syndrome however, it is an autosomal recessive disorder due to cystathionine B-synthetase deficiency. Elevated levels of homocystine, homocystine metabolites and methionine accumulate in blood and urine. The urinary excess of these substances may be identified by a positive cyanide nitroprusside test, but the diagnosis is based upon urine and plasma amino acid analysis. The diagnosis may be further confirmed by studies of cystathionine B-synthetase activity in a liver biopsy specimen. Similar to Marfan syndrome, major manifestations of homocystinuria are found in the skeletal system, the vascular system, and the eye. Additionally, between one-third and three-quarters of untreated homocystinurics have mild to moderate mental retardation.

Untreated patients display dolichostenomelia, arachnodactyly, pectus carinatum or excavatum, kyphoscoliosis, and dental malalignment. Radiographs may

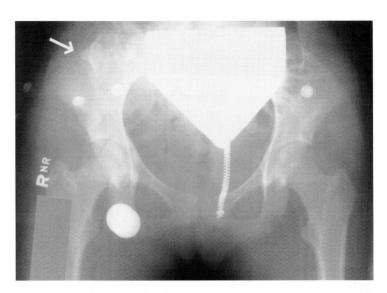

Figure 7.6. Iliac horn extruding from ilium.

Figure 7.7. Small hypoplastic patella.

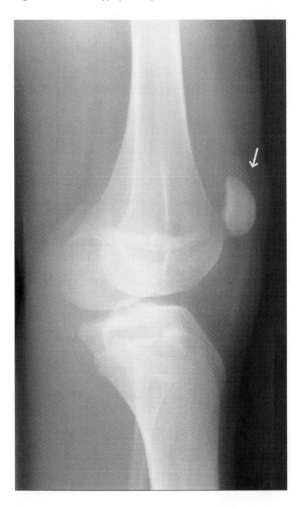

additionally show osteoporosis and bioconcave vertebral bodies. The vascular problems associated with homocystinuria are arterial and venous thromboembolic phenomena. Myopia and ectopia lentis are also characteristic findings in homocystinuria. The lens displacement in homocystinuria is typically downward. Because of the clinical overlap, homocystinuria should be ruled out by blood and urine biochemical testing in patients who show the phenotypic characteristics common in Marfan syndrome and homocystinuria.

Nail–patella syndrome

The diagnostic quartet characteristic of the nail–patella syndrome consists of dystrophic nails, absent or hypoplastic patellae, defects of the elbow, and iliac "horns." The disorder is autosomal dominant, due to a mutation in the LMX1B gene located at chromosome 9q34. The principal clinical manifestations of the nail–patella syndrome are found in the nails, in the skeletal system, and in the kidney. Nail changes are almost always identifiable at birth. They include longitudinal ridging or splitting and in some instances, absence of a portion or all of a nail (anonychia). Iliac "horns" are not known to occur in any other disorder in humans or in any other primates, and are therefore pathognomonic for this disorder. These iliac "horns" are posterior central iliac exostoses that are identifiable in 80 percent of patients with nail–patella syndrome (Figure 7.6). At the elbow, there is capitellar dysplasia, and the radial head is generally dislocated posteriorly with accompanying cubitus valgus. There is diminished forearm rotation, as well as extension block of the elbow. The patellae are hypoplastic or absent, and there is significant genu valgum, which tends to be progressive resulting in patellar subluxation and dislocation (Figures 7.7 & 7.8) and often requiring surgical management. Other musculoskeletal abnormalities include a stiff valgus hindfoot, stiffness of the distal finger joints, clinodactyly of the fifth digit, a

Figure 7.8. Dislocated patella.

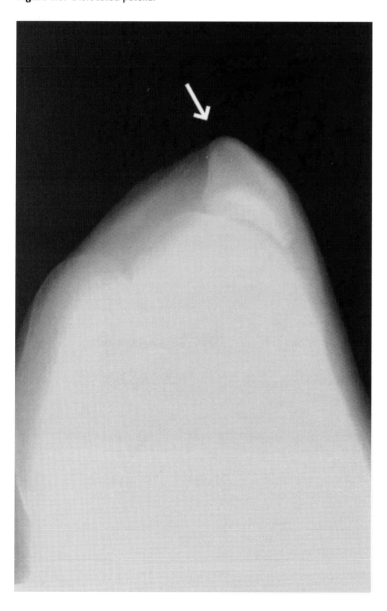

Table 7.1 *List of selected skeletal dysplasias with associated gene abnormality*

Gene	Skeletal dysplasia type
Collagen	
COL1A1	Osteogenesis imperfecta types I–IV
COL2A1	Hypochondroplasia
	Spondyloepiphyseal dysplasia (SED) congenita
	Spondyloepimetaphyseal dysplasia (SEMD)
Fibroblast growth factor receptor	
FGFR2	Apert syndrome
FGFR3	Achondroplasia
Other	
Fibrillin 1	Marfan syndrome
PHEX gene	X-linked hypophosphatemic rickets
EVC gene	Ellis–van Creveld syndrome
LMX1B	Nail–patella syndrome
COMP (cartilage oligomeric protein)	Pseudoachondroplasis multiple epiphyseal dysplasia (Fairbank and Ribbing types)
DTDST (diastrophic dysplasia sulfate transporter)	Diastrophic dysplasia
SOX9	Camptomelic dysplasia
Sedlin gene	Spondyloepiphyseal dysplasia tarda
Arylsulfatase E	Chondrodysplasia punctata
EBP (CDXD)	X-linked dominant chondrodysplasia punctata (Conradi–Hunermann)
ARSE (Arylsulfatase A)	Chondrodysplasia punctata (brachytelephalangic)
PEX 7	Rhizomelic chondrodysplasia punctata
PEX1, PEX2, PEX5, PEX6	Chondrodysplasia punctata (Zellweger syndrome)
IDA gene (alpha-1-iduronidase)	Mucopolysaccharidosis (MPS I)
DIS gene (iduronate-2-sulfatase)	Mucopolysaccharidosis II (MPS II)
GALNS (Galactose-6-sulfatase)	Mucopolysaccharidosis IVA (MPS IVA)
GLBI (beta-galactosidase)	Mucopolysaccharidosis IVB (MPS IVB)
EXT1 gene (exostosin-1)	Multiple exostoses
EXT2 gene (exostosin-2)	Multiple exostoses
EXT3 gene (exostosin-30	Multiple exostoses

prominent outer clavicle, scoliosis, and abnormalities of the pectoralis minor, biceps, triceps, and quadriceps muscles.

Renal disease findings are present in approximately 50 percent of patients. The degree of renal involvement varies both within and between families. The most frequent symptoms of renal disease are proteinuria, hematuria, and hypertension. Renal concentrating ability may be impaired. Electron microscope changes on renal biopsy may be pathognomonic. Due to the frequency of clinically significant orthopedic difficulties, orthopedic consultation is recommended (Table 7.1).

Index